A STROKE OF BAD LUCK

*Reconditioning Mind and Body
for a New and Rewarding Lifestyle*

by Sebastiaan Bakker

A Stroke of Bad Luck
An Autobiography

Published by DH Publishing
First published 2012

Table of Contents

Table of Illustrations

Disclaimer

The information found in this book is not intended to be a substitute for professional medical advice. One should not use this information to either diagnose or treat a health-problem and/or disease without first consulting with a qualified health-care provider. Please consult a medical specialist with any questions or concerns you may have regarding your condition. The charts in this book provide an indication of progress of recovery by the author over time. There is no scientific support to the percentages and time-frame. Based on subjective data, they solely illustrate the author's perception. The curves in the charts will differ for each individual. Despite the lack of scientific value, the author believes that his illustrations and the accompanying text can help others to make their own assessment with respect to recovery.

Acknowledgement

To my wife Dorthe, my two sons, Sven and Henrik, and my family and friends. I owe you my life for all the love, care and patience that I received

To the professional personnel of Ullevål Universitets Sykehus, Diakonhjemmet Sykehus, Sunnaas Rehabiliterings Sykehus, Cato Senteret, Rikshopspitalet, Centrum Logopedi, and my personal trainers

Finally yet importantly, to all the people who have suffered a brain stroke and their friends and family—that they may benefit from the experience that I have gained and try to share by telling my story

Foreword

Brain strokes are all different and without discrimination of sex, age, or physical condition. We share one common objective: reconditioning the mind and body for new and rewarding lifestyles, however different that may turn out to be. I hope that I can contribute to a better understanding of what it takes to recover and make it easier for others to draw their own plan or place their situation in perspective.

Like so many things in life, recovery is not something that happens overnight. Unless you believe in miracles, nothing is free in this world. You have to work hard and long to create your own miracles. Accept all the support you can get. Leave no room for negative thoughts. The power of positive thinking is the key to successful rehabilitation. The reward at the end of the adventure of rehabilitation is enormous. The experience made me humble and appreciative of the small things in life. Although uncalled for, that is not a bad thing.

How Your World Changes

Dorthe and I had celebrated our seventh wedding anniversary with a splendid dinner in downtown Oslo. We had sold our house in the Netherlands a few years earlier. After we had left for Norway, the country where my wife Dorthe came from, we had lived at a number of fine-looking places along the Oslo fjord. Our plans were nearing completion: leaving the short but striking summers and long cold winters behind to live aboard a sailboat in the Mediterranean—at least for a few years until we were ready to settle in a place that we had not yet decided upon. Our talks kept ending on the same topics: the well-being of our two sons—Sven and Henrik—now old enough to look after themselves, and the practical arrangements we would have to make. In anticipation of the change, we had rented a waterfront apartment and further reduced our inventory as we had done during our previous moves.

Drowsily I sat up in my bed; the room was still in total darkness. My sense of orientation had totally vanished. The space I knew so well was gone. Reasoning with myself, I started my

1

search for the exit; there had to be a door somewhere! In the murky room, I quietly shuffled forward: my hands softly tapping the wall. I stumbled into the furniture and a table lamp crashed on the floor. Awakened by the noise, Dorthe flipped on her reading light. The moment she saw my desperation, her irritation with the violent awakening melted. I was totally lost, and she knew that something was terribly wrong. "It's my brain…my brain. Call an ambulance!" I called out, and my body collapsed. Not much later, I was at Ullevål Sykehus.

Strangely enough, at the hospital I remained conscious up to the point where the doctors completed their diagnosis. The blood stream to the brain was blocked. It led to a stroke in the brain stem, which manages the body's biological stability and the basic life support systems. It is easier to describe what still worked after the stroke than vice versa. Swallowing was without reaction; my eyesight distorted the surroundings; I fell when trying to stand; one side of my body was without feeling; limbs would not move without meditation; my voice was hardly a whisper. The only thing that still worked was my breathing. From there to eternity was a small step. The neurologist was not sure that I would last another night. Intensive care took over. I did not fight for my life; neither did the medics. There was no hectic running or shouting. The verdict was not mine. My brain had to resume control on its own.

Sven flew in from Amsterdam on the first flight. Henrik arrived immediately after Dorthe had broken the news to him. Our sons were present at the hospital during the first days, and within a matter of weeks, they became frequent flyers. Both of them lived in the Netherlands: Henrik studying in The Hague; Sven, running his own business in the Amsterdam area. I remember that I was afraid to upset Henrik's studies while he was in the midst of his exams. Already before landing in intensive care, I had told Dorthe not to alarm him unnecessarily. I believed in survival. Instinct knows no rationale. Little do I remember of the days that followed. I lived by the color of emotions: love, trust, and safety. Not until afterward did Dorthe and the boys brief me on the details. For a long time, we did not speak of those dreadful days burdened with fear.

The neurologist's uncertainty slowly turned into a cautious confidence. After a few days, I was moved to a regular hospital room to begin my healing. My survival seemingly secured; the worst was behind me; yet, I did not know what was coming.

Dorthe communicated every bit of news to the outside world. It was wearing her out physically and mentally, but she saw it as her duty to keep many personally informed. Fortunately, the tam-tam sounded before she buckled under the effort. Dorthe kept Sven and Henrik, my younger brother, and her parents up-to-date. The people she spoke to made sure that the intelligence spread through the family tree. My closest family and friends were there for me. The mental support of their visits was essential, even when I was only half-conscious; my existence was confirmed in the glance at the people I cared for. Their quiet presence mattered.

Maybe I am just being naïve or it may be part of the instinctive survival mechanism, but from day one there has never been any doubt about making it—although Dorthe and I never dared to qualify the state that I could be in long term. We did not discuss that topic until the "medical emergencies" showed signs of recovery. Both of us silently decided that we would live with the limitations that could not be restored; as inconveniences, we banned them from our thoughts. What we had done was to separate the important functions that needed full attention from the trivial shortcomings. The short list created itself and kept changing thereafter. It gave us a clear view of priorities. For stabilizing my biological and life support functions, I had an easy job; I was totally dependent on others.

I had lost my first wife Mil and Sven his mother when he was fourteen. What started as breast cancer had ended with a fatal brain tumor. I was all he had left of his parents, and I felt his sorrow and fear when he recognized similar symptoms in me that he had seen in his mother. I had to recover. Failure was not an option. "Please, do not let us down—for the need to love," I pleaded.

One of the things that I had admired so much in Mil was her attitude in the final phase of her life. She left no room for negative thoughts—never, not even the simplest of complaints. All her willpower and energy were directed at making the best out of the time she had left. Mil refused to mentally retire prematurely. Nobody would suffer more from the loss of the remains of life than she would. Mil had decided to be open about her situation with family and friends. As always, she was straightforward and did not hide anything from the world—not even her loss of hair: "There is nothing worse than people whispering behind your back not knowing if they are supposed to know. Nobody gains anything unless they can talk to you." A positive mind-set protected her joy for life. She shared what she radiated, and her last lesson was an immense gift.

Would I be strong enough to do the same? From above, Mil was looking over me as my guardian angel and concurring with my parents; she would give me a helping hand in desperate times. Down on earth, Dorthe, Sven and Henrik, my family at large, and our dear friends would pull me through.

4

Getting Out of the Doldrums

Ullevål Sykehus was typical for an older hospital downtown. Despite the modern hallways, the original architectural details of the main building were distinct: tiled corridors, vain protrusions, high ceilings, and the acoustics of a mausoleum. With age came the medical expertise of the nearby university. Fortunately, I had a place for myself where visitors could not disturb other patients during off hours—when my hiccups played up or when I had fun with the boys. My wheelchair was parked between my bed and a small desk; in the corner, there was a sink with a mirror. I had to laugh when Sven could not resist a balancing act on just two wheels in my means of local transport. In case I would ever need a driving instructor, we could keep it in the family. Good-humored, the kids pulled out their cell phones for a photo shoot. With my black eye patch, I looked like a retired pirate with the youngsters hanging over my shoulder as colorful parrots. We had fun in spite of troubled times, and that was worth a lot to all of us.

Although it was a room with a view over the old complex with its beautiful high trees, most of the time the thick curtains were drawn. My eyes did not favor the direct sunlight. The lines of the moldings along the ceiling deformed the space. Double vision made me tired. Wearing an eye patch only partly solved the problem. Eventually my lazy eye would have to face the reality of practical training.

It was one of those mornings where everything seemed possible. For the first time in a long time, I felt well rested after a good night's sleep. The nurses smiled, and empty coffee cups rattled in the corridor. There was an inexplicable brilliance to the lively morning chatter. Tall windows let in the light of a sparkling daybreak. The air was different today.

This was a day for change. I had grown a short beard and longed for a wet shave. An unshaven look may be fashionable, but not today. One of the nurses volunteered to do the job. "No, thank you. If you help me across the room and hand me my shaving kit, I would like to give it a try," I replied. Four eyes stared back at me from above the sink. It took me an hour to complete what is normally a five-minute morning routine. The brain startled with the mirrored image; my pose, coordination, touch, and eyesight sabotaged pulling the blade. Whatever way you look at it, I had underestimated the effort or overestimated my ability. I came out undamaged; the triumph was mine. I was on my way back to being self-sufficient. However small the step, I had something to be proud of and smiled broadly. To feel good, it helps to look good. The fresh feeling boosted my self-esteem.

That October, spring was in the air. "Would you like to shower, or shall I wash you here in bed?" the nurse asked. I eagerly accepted her first offer. Although I was unaware of what I had said yes to, she wheeled me a couple of doors down the hall into what could have been a mini car wash. Sitting in a plastic chair, one side of my body felt the hot water hitting me like ice-cold needles; the steamy atmosphere made me gasp for air. It took my mind and body time to agree on the conflicting sensations. After a few more suspicious attempts, the cascade of hot water became an agreeable experience. Dorthe was waiting for me when I entered the room in clean, ironed pajamas. Her astonished look made me feel a hundred times better than the change in appearance: "You look fantastic; unbelievable!" she cheered. For a moment, the "look and feel" suppressed the complexity of the situation. In between, the nurses had changed the bed linen; it was white and crispy. I felt like a prince.

The first month passed without my real involvement. Nurses and doctors did what they do best. I submitted myself to their daily agenda and was wheeled from one test to another. Discussions went mostly over my head. Not that it mattered much. My level of comprehension was not up to speed to participate. On top of that, being a Dutchman, my Norwegian was inadequate, which made it problematic to express myself. My contribution was limited to a physical presence. I trusted my partner and hospital staff. Dorthe had taken on the role of interpreter. Without any limits to her "power of attorney," she dealt with all decisions, communications, and practical arrangements. I was very lucky to have her by my side.

The kindness and dedication of the nurses was striking. If not already offered, nothing seemed too much to ask. Despite their skilled efficiency, their approach was always delicate and personal. My guests were treated equally hospitably, which cleared the inevitable tension of a hospital call. Unable to look after even the simplest of things myself, I felt humble to encounter such goodness. I found peace with my dependency. Although there was not much that I could physically do, I sought out my contributions as a member of the team; being a good patient was one of them. Whereas doctors and nurses receive years of education, the patient is not trained for being subjected to the situation. Becoming a patient is something overwhelming that suddenly happens to you. Unprepared, people end up in a hospital bed. From personal experience I say, "Give it the best of your attitude, a smile, and a 'thank you;' it will not go unrewarded."

Being short of comprehension and awareness relieved me of unnecessary stress. Underestimating the severity of the situation might be ignorant, but that is irrelevant. A positive way of looking at it is to view it as a valuable defense mechanism. Being unable to control the outcome forced me to surrender to the priority of resting without the worry of the moment or the future. Knowing that you are in good hands is crucial.

It took a month to get me in the medical safe zone. Swallowing was still not possible, but the fastidious feeding directly into my stomach finally worked. Slowly, I had become more and more aware of my surroundings and the people around me. It marked the end of my stay at Ullevål Sykehus. My next stop was Diakonhjemmet Sykehus, where the medics would attend to detail. My task was widening the confines of a new life.

As much as I was afraid of the answer, I could no longer hold up my curiosity. "Will my old self return one day? How long does it take to recover?" I asked pryingly when parting. I should have known better. Doctors possess a form of hesitant diplomacy when it comes to giving their prognosis. It is in their DNA. I cannot blame them for not giving me a straightforward answer—certainly not for avoiding the risk of a setback in my motivation. It was unfair to put them on the spot. Statistics are the only valid source of reference for specialists to predict an outcome. Dots on a scatter diagram may be mathematically interesting, but there is only one of me.

For a start, my question was wrong—or at least too broad to answer. How do you define recovery, and to which extent or in what time frame? There are too many pieces in the puzzle to be conclusive. A rewarding life, despite potential disabilities, is something very private. In that respect, mental strength matters more than physical abilities. Even under similar conditions, personal drive makes all the difference. I realized that the answer lay inside of me. Yes, I can, with will-power and a positive mind-set, coach my revival; recovery is a fluid endeavor without retort.

The functions of the little brain and brain stem are explained in layman's terms. In simple words, a disorder resulting from a stroke in that part of the brain may affect your well-being and functioning. For the benefit to the medically illiterate reader, I will avoid the use of neurological jargon. As a result, the synopsis lacks the professional exactitude normally exercised among specialists.

The primary function of the little brain is to integrate information provided by the body's sensors and to coordinate the actions to maintain balance and control movements. To that purpose, it includes processing the overwhelming stream of neural data of the feedback system. If, as a result of a stroke, that system is in disarray, it destabilizes the ability to master fine movements and maintain our posture and balance, and it may impact the aptitude to relearn. Muscular strength is often affected by a stroke in the little brain. It obscures the recovery visibly. In addition, modern research supports the role of the little brain in cognitive functions, including attention, language, music, and time.

The brain stem is the lower part of the brain and joins the little brain with the spinal cord. The brain stem is small but vital. Most of the neural information between brain and body passes through the hundreds of millions of nerve connections it contains. This includes a wealth of signals pertaining to motor functions, crude and fine touch, vibrations, itching, pain, temperature, and body-part orientation. As the brain stem also polices the central nervous system, it is in command of the state of consciousness and controls the sleep cycle. Most crucial is the role of the brain stem in regulating the pulse and breathing. If that function permanently fails, it is game over.

My First Steps to Recovery

Diakonhjemmet Sykehus, wedged between Slemdalsveien and Sørkedalsveien, is a relatively small hospital in Oslo. Although part of Norway's government-controlled health system, it is still managed by a foundation. Over time, the original Christian character lost its dominance, but the norms and values remained outspoken; angels have replaced the nuns.

Today, the hospital is best described as personal, friendly, and service-minded. It lacks the appearance of administrative efficiency that one finds on the campus of large medical institutions. It has intimacy. It was the perfect place to recover after the first few weeks of intensive medical treatment at Ullevål Sykehus. The doctors and nurses at Diakonhjemmet were excellent, and so were their therapists of various disciplines. I experienced an understanding of my needs that was unique. I would be their guest for the next two months.

The welcome by Nina was warm and personal. She assigned me a double room with the standard outfitting of cabinets, a washbasin, an overhead TV, the usual medical control panel,

11

and space to park my wheelchair. Visiting hours existed but were hardly adhered to—as long as you respected the privacy of your neighbors and did not obstruct the staff. Down the corridor was a simple lounge with seating arrangements, newspapers, and a large-screen television set. People used the space to meet their visitors, watch the news, or eat and chat a little with fellow patients. During my stay, I appreciated that living room more and more. After the morning routine, Dorthe or one of the nurses would take me there in my wheelchair with a tripod with plasma and nutrition in its wake. It was nice to get out of bed, see other people, and be active. Socialization is an important aspect of rehabilitation. Being part of the world brought back the "can-do" attitude: more and more, little by little.

Dorthe was a teacher; in addition to me, she had a hundred-plus students to look after. Nonetheless, she would visit en route to work. Those early stopovers were brief, not more than a quarter of an hour, but marked the start of a new day with a morning kiss.After a day of work at the fashion academy, she would return in the evening to spend quality time with me. I would demonstrate the records I had broken, flip through the pages of my notebook in which I had practiced my handwriting, show off my footwork, watch a movie, and secretly nibble on a piece of fluffy cake that Dorthe brought. We made the best out of it, but it is not easy to remain one entity when separated.

I had work to do...not much...but demanding...enough to force me into frequent rests. Instead of enjoying a time-out, I hated the weekends. My trainers had their well-deserved breaks; to my impatience, rehabilitation was on hold. Those days were long and irritating. "Snap out of it," was Dorthe's proverb whenever I gave in to self-pity or trapped myself in a loop of mental circles around something insignificant. Still today, she puts me straight with her "Snap out of it" when that happens. It helps, because I know that she is right. Handling stress was once my stronghold, but now I easily lose myself. Once one clumsy thing gets loaded on top of another and another, there seems no end to it. Unless I distance myself and start from scratch, it will not get any better.

The first steps to recovery were inspiring. During the months at Diakonhjemmet Sykehus, the therapists worked mostly on my swallowing, mobility, and coordination. The changes did not happen overnight. It took weeks of training, but the efforts paid off. I still faced limitations, but with caution, I could eat and drink, move around, and perform the basic personal chores. On the medical chart, I went from 'intermittent' to 'steady.' Approvingly, the hospital staff watched my progress. My reward was a weekend leave.

Dorthe packed the dirty laundry and folded the wheelchair in the trunk, and we drove off as soon as we could—soon, not fast. At the first roundabout off the premises, things went wrong. "Slow down; stop!" I screamed. The car seemed to be rolling over. I was holding onto the dashboard, armrest, seat, and ceiling—anything I could grab as the car seemed to tumble. It seemed ages before the panic disappeared, and I fell back in the passenger seat. "Breathe…breathe…control your breathing." I kept repeating this to myself and gazed at Dorthe. She had stopped the car alongside the curb of the roundabout; the orange emergency lights were flashing in the darkness. Slowly my bewilderment faded. Head up, I recovered from a total loss of orientation.

Oslo had seen little snow that winter; the lights seemed dimmed by the absence of a white reflection of the streets.

Without a fix on any sighting, my feel for up or down had gone astray. The slight inclination of the car in the curve had triggered the perceived roll. It was an unforeseen complication. Dorthe flicked off the panic lights. Slowly, she pulled out and guided me home by an artificial horizon. "Left turn ahead; straight at the roundabout, and speeding up." She forewarned as an experienced navigator. From now on, car travel was restricted to daytime.

Our home was a unique fit to the situation. The elevator went straight up from the parking garage in the basement to our apartment; there was no hassle with mud, snow, and ice. I could wheel myself right up to the front door. With everything ground floor and no thresholds, it was easy to get around. I was home among the warmth of our own interior—a bottle of wine and two glasses waiting on the table and flowers everywhere. That evening, Dorthe served me a gourmet welcome-home dinner: small tartars of fresh seafood that were rich in taste and easy to swallow. Here I could invite our friends again but equally easy excuse myself for a short nap or to turn in early.

Whatever the weather, Dorthe would take me outside for a tour along the Herbern Marina or push me downtown for an espresso in one of the small cafés off Stortingsgata. It was not my return to society yet, but it was a huge step in the right direction.

I longed to be part of the large family gathering for Christmas. Spending the holidays in everybody's company would mean much to me. In line with family traditions, we would come together in her parents' vacation home in Sweden. I loved the people and the simplicity of the place. Compared to this, the outlook of an uneventful week in a deserted hospital was not very appealing. The Christmas tree in the community room was not going to change that. On the contrary, the decorations and Christmas carols on the radio made my desire even stronger.

The tune of Chris Rea's lyrics kept playing in my head:

> Driving home for Christmas
> Oh, I can't wait to see those faces
> I'm driving home for Christmas, yea
> Well I'm moving down that line
> And it's been so long
> But I will be there.

I wanted out; I needed to break away from sickbay for a few days to recharge my batteries. My rehabilitation was scheduled to begin in the new year. The crossover from medical to physical recovery called for a different kind of energy. I was in search of a milestone to mark the change from a passive to an active regime.

Dorthe's dad was hesitant to make any promises of celebrating the holidays in their house in the Swedish forest. The remoteness of the place in case of a medical emergency worried him; there was always the risk of being snowed-in. It was his decision to make. I respected his judgment. Meeting my nutritional needs was straightforward. The blender would do an excellent job of mashing the traditional dishes beyond recognition and making them easy to swallow. My desire created the extra drive. There was little time left to prove to him that I could be a low-risk guest: an asset, however small, not a liability. Strong desires are strong motivators.

I had worked my way down to the cafeteria off the entrance hall to meet him halfway. Despite my pajamas, nothing seemed overtly wrong; relaxed, we enjoyed our sodas and chatted. That same evening he called Dorthe. "The family Christmas is on!" he said. What had made him change his mind was the sudden realization of the speed at which I had improved during those long weeks preceding Christmas.

Physical recovery is not something to consider as long as the life support system and biological stability is in total disarray. When discharged from the medical hospitals to go into rehabilitation, I had partially recovered my independence. I could use the restroom on my own, dress myself, eat at the dinner table, and get around by myself. Little by little, my capability to comprehend, evaluate, and communicate came back in my daily life.

Occasionally the path of recovery was overcome by emotion. I shed tears of gratitude and joy along the road. My fragile sentiment was no match for many of the strong sensations. My feelings got the upper hand when I shuffled through the corridor without contact to the handrail, when I overcame my fear of going up and down the stairs, or finished my first serving. It created a bond with the therapists. The harder the patient works for it, the higher the incentive for the trainer; the accomplishments are the result of a shared effort. Rehabilitation is something very personal. One thing is for sure: it cannot be delegated.

Find Inner Strength

I took my camera and waded through the thick layer of snow to the edge of the terrace; the tripod made a good walking aid. The light was dramatic; shades of orange and purple stretched over the southwestern sky. End-of-day colors reflected on the giant ice flakes. Off the coast, a cold fisherman pulled his nets slowly through the icy water with silent seagulls in its wake. I had to work fast; it was almost four o'clock. The light changes rapidly in the north. I had to grasp the moment before it was gone.

With the camera in front of me on the stand, I examined the myriad of settings. I had bought the camera just before I ended up in the hospital but only now had time to study the functions. The directions of use were in fine print. It was my first confrontation with complexity in a long time. I read, re-read, and pounded over the meaning repeatedly before it made sense. My brain and eyesight almost buckled under the effort. Eventually I locked in my final adjustments. Facing the sunset, high up on the eastern flank of the fjord, the nature is pure and present. The pictures captured the enormity of what I had felt on the rooftop of Sunnaas Sykehus.

Sunnaas Sykehus combines the dignity of a sanatorium with functional simplicity. It is a world-renowned rehabilitation center. Tokens of appreciation from all over the world proudly testify to its reputation. The founders, the Sunnaas couple Rolf and Birgit, were ahead of their time. Empathy—along with genuineness and positive regard—is the pillar of their success. Sunnaas Sykehus combines that quality with service-minded people, knowledge, and the soothing beauty of nature.

People congratulated me with the admission. Diakonhjemmet Sykehus had worked hard on following up on the application; I was granted the maximum of a three-month stay. The ambience was surprisingly positive: no subdued hospital atmosphere. Front desk had been expecting my arrival. Dorthe was treated to a friendly smile and a professional welcome; the cook stepped out of his kitchen with two muffins and introduced himself, eager to make me feel at home.

Suppertime was ridiculously early. It took some getting used to; then again, when in Rome, do as the Romans do. The further north you go, the earlier people take their evening meal: Rome at ten, Amsterdam at six, and Oslo at five, while, on the other side of the world, people have breakfast. My discomfort was not just a matter of my biological clock or cultural differences. The late-afternoon dinners made my evenings dreadfully long. Having many hours left in the day is great for some, but to me it was annoying. With the gym and pool closed, it was a waste of valuable time and attractive resources. I was here on a mission. Hanging out in front of the TV to kill time before I could eventually turn in was not going to further my recovery.

I worked as if physically and mentally unbreakable to get most out of my stay. Smiles, compliments, and approving looks fueled my motivation. I was proud of my achievements and shared that pride with whomever wanted a piece. The evenings still young, I wandered through the deserted corridors, climbed the stairs relentlessly, and did my balancing act on one foot until I tipped—only to try again and again. I explored the maze of hallways...deeper and deeper...longer and longer. "Dr. Livingstone, I presume," one joked. I had discovered a new and happy tribe in a different sector. The patients here had other disabilities. Mentally sound and energetic, they were having a good time. Their playful good spirit amazed me.

Not all training has to be guided by therapists. I strongly believe in repetition. That, I could do on my own. Awareness of my limitations inspired the creation of new exercises. Opportunities to practice are available wherever you look. You just have to grab them. It takes time to reprogram the brain to act on autopilot. Years go by before a child masters all of his functions smoothly. Through curiosity and play, mistakes and corrections, infants learn and progress. I had one advantage: I had knowledge of the route and the ultimate destination. I also had a disadvantage: I had to find the child in me.

Morning gymnastics were fun. They were a pleasant way to wake up mind and muscles. Jokingly, we helped each other out as we maneuvered across our soft-matted playground to loosen up and play ball. It made a friendly start, always respecting each other's abilities and tempo; it set the tone of the house. Speech, swallowing, occupational therapy, mending my eyesight, and creative balance exercises filled my days. If not lead, they were self-imposed. Learning was not restricted to indoor training. Short rounds on the grounds with Nordic walking sticks offered clean air and fresh snow.

I could easily keep up with the group. The others never waited impatiently for me to catch up. The truth lay in an unusual combination of an all-embracing, but still distant, social attitude. Nobody would ever get too far ahead or show intolerance—neither verbally, nor through body language. The subtle sense of protecting the motivation and privacy of others was constantly present. We took care of each other, not medically or domestically, but with a smile, a kind word, and questions of genuine interest. People had enough to deal with to get too close. Still, after a few months, you got to know each other a little bit better. For most, I have a deep respect for the way they managed themselves and their personal drive to get better.

Whenever Dorthe bumped into the staff, they never held back on their raving reviews. Made eager by their enthusiasm, she ran past me in order to see me showing off my latest achievements. I had been waiting for her in the lobby. By the time I got up, she was already halfway to my room. They stimulated Dorthe's sentiment; she got ahead of herself.

Dorthe drove me from Sunnaas to Ullevål Sykehus for medical tests. Traces of dirty snow, protected by deep shadows, marked the blindingly wet country road. In the low sun, crocuses took over the fresh space. Just the two of us touring the landscape in warmth and privacy was happiness. For both of us, making the trip had meant taking the day off. I enjoyed the mini vacation.

We confiscated a cafeteria table in the lobby for some refreshments. Dorthe was halfway toward the counter to place the order when she ran into the neurologist who had taken me under his wings as I had arrived half a year ago. I saw them talk a little and point at me. I recognized him too, got up, and walked over to say hello. We will never forget the look on his face when I shook his hand: total disbelief as if he saw water burning. He never expected my recovery to have worked out so well. In amazement, he called to mind my critical days in intensive care. He did not have to comment on my rehabilitation, nor did I expect a free consultation in the lobby; I was no longer his patient. We exchanged a few more words after which he apologized and hurried toward the elevator to join his shift on a new working day. The broad smile on his face told me I had made his day worthwhile. It worked both ways; I was on the right track, and he had put me there.

Time had come to move on to my next stop at CATO Senteret in the coastal town of Son. A nurse offered the opportunity of taking a break. "Spend some weeks at home," She suggested. I was used to being away during the week. I knew that as soon as I disrupted the rhythm of rehabilitation, it would be hard to pick it up again. Right or wrong, I moved on without hesitation and without a break. It took time to adjust to the change. At Sunnaas Sykehus, the focus had been on restoring specific functions. The therapists had worked with me one-on-one. CATO Senteret did little of that. Their's was a collective approach. Amidst the crowd, I missed a thumbs-up. I felt lonely. I was so close to completing my rehabilitation but so far away from home…and even further from a return to society.

CATO Senteret is like a three-star theme hotel. The rooms, reception area, and restaurant were an exact replica of a family hotel; training and outdoor events represented the theme. No uniforms for the hardly visible employees, buffet servings with free seating, and fixed hours for activities advertised on the billboard; I was in a different world, not my world. They tried to make me a guest by pretending to be a hotel, but the makeover lacked a smile and personal attentiveness. It was an unusual transformation attempt and depressive in a peculiar way. Then again, I was here on business.

I could have easily overslept; there was no safety net of nurses to check on me. Setting the alarm was my own responsibility. I missed the familiar faces and people I had bonded with, the white-uniformed personnel that would answer my questions, and my place at the dinner table; empathy had vanished. The rehabilitation philosophy was very different from what I had grown accustomed to. At CATO Senteret, I was forced to take back control over my life: from getting up, to turning in, and everything in between. It took time to realize their intentions. The goal of CATO Senteret is to prepare their guests for self-sufficiency in day-to-day life. The approach is subtly confrontational; the atmosphere, somewhat deceptive. I had always embraced change. If not imposed by others, I would proclaim it myself. But now the flexibility to do so had left me. My brain was rigidly holding on to the routine of the old regime. Here, I had to face and overcome the challenges of my physical and mental limitations. Once the expectations became clear, I regained my stance, and things turned to the better.

Cato Zahl Pedersen, one of the founders of CATO Senteret, is a national hero. He won over a dozen gold medals, explored the Antarctic, and mountaineered the roof of the world. The man is extraordinary; his accomplishments are despite an accident which cost him both his arms in his childhood. He is a rehabilitation expert through personal experience. His over-performance is rooted in psychological conditioning. Commitment, courage, and willpower form the foundation of his successful endeavors. This modern Viking rejected the boundaries of his possibilities; not "Impossible" but "I'm possible" is his motto. His drive appealed to me. My ambitions differed, but Cato Zahl confirmed my personal and professional beliefs.

His thinking was inspiring. I enjoyed his speech for the rehabilitants. His take on many of the issues was concise: "You cannot control destiny, but do take charge when it comes to dealing with it. Focus on what you have, not on what you have lost. Negative thoughts are limiting; positive thoughts create possibilities." He continued. His aim is to help people find fulfillment in their lives upon returning to society by fostering the will to change with goal setting, determination, motivation, and teamwork. CATO Senteret reflects his ideas in their approach. The therapies were mostly aimed at fine-tuning what was already set in motion at Sunnaas Sykehus. The biggest contribution was coaching me to rely on my inner strength to regain control.

The exercise leader did more than her best—as if on stage with Ricky Martin at a rock-concert. The small pack could not follow her complex choreography and wavered along rhythmlessly. Her movements were too advanced. I did not need to fail. I put my shoes on, tied them, and left the room. At times, one has to protect one's motivation, but I felt the effect for days. Without the occasional eye contact and empathy, personal consideration is easily lost in group sessions. At times, I felt overlooked. Still, it is a fair representation of what I could expect when making my re-entry into society.

Rehabilitation is a test of character. The stay at CATO Senteret strengthened my defensibility. I was nearing the end of my formal rehabilitation track but had not fully regained my mental independence. At home, I would have to continue laboring my physical and mental potency. Nine months had gone by; it was time to test my renewed skills in the real world.

Under My Own Steam

Our dream had vaporized before leaving port. A second chance seemed far out of reach. We did not waste our energy on the disappointment. One day we would mill over new plans; after all, dreams are the spice of life. First, we had to explore the horizon of a new realism. For that, I had to get better...much better.

We had to get our life back. Dorthe and I needed to regain equal footing and excitement in our marriage. In our Oslo apartment, we lived mostly indoors. The layout and location was an excellent match for my capability. Dorthe had given up her job to be with me. Due to—or despite—the conveniences, there was an immovable emptiness. We lacked a thrill in our lives. The idea of breaking away from dull routines and another long demanding Norwegian winter was growing on us. A sabbatical could change that. The freedom to do so was at hand.

Dorthe and I forced a radical change of environment upon us. We decided to move to the south of Spain on the

Mediterranean coast. On the Internet, it was easy to find a one-year lease. A few e-mails later, we signed for a simple town house with a small front yard and a back garden. Our new residence was within walking distance to the port of Puerto Banus with its super-yachts, shops, restaurants, and lovely beaches. Although ashore, it resembled our original dream of living aboard a sailboat.

We left Oslo in a car that was stuffed with what it could hold, and that would be it for the year. It was astonishing how little we actually needed. We took only the most "vital" things: Dorthe's sewing machine, my laptop, the espresso machine, the accessories, sporting goods, and clothes for the beach and a stylish evening out. Years earlier, we had moved from the Netherlands to Oslo with two containers of cargo. Now we moved again with nothing more than some bits and pieces. We never missed what was left behind. Material possessions were not going to make us happy. Going back to basics was a refreshing experience. It made it easier to focus on what was important in life.

The Costa del Sol is a popular vacation destination throughout the year. For the most part, the available accommodations are second homes. The setting turned out to be more international than traditional Spanish. After all, enjoying each other's company had priority. Our temporary home was less than an hour's drive from Malaga airport. It was unproblematic to find a budget airline to the region. Our children and friends made frequent use of the easy flight connections; we could take pleasure in their presence, share our good fortune, and offer them a good time that was easy on the pocketbook. We were never alone for long. As simple as it was for others to join us in the south, it was trouble-free for us to revisit the Nordic.

The al fresco lifestyle is very social. Most of life in the warm summer and mild winter of lovely Marbella happened outdoors. We enjoyed the many new friends. Fifi, Dorthe's girlfriend from next door, helped us to find our way around. We took turns hosting neighbors for a glass of wine and shared dinners. Forgotten domestic chores and pleasures became part of life again: working in the garden, washing the car, food shopping, and trying out regional recipes. I intensified my fitness training. Spain provided an excellent setting for outdoor exercising. Almost daily, we toured on our mountain bikes. Spending time in the sun at the pool or while sightseeing was a welcome diversion, without which, life would be all work and no play. Life offers more than the constant analyses of how you perform when trying to be somewhat useful.

The white flowers of the Dame de Noche released a heavy perfume. Hortensia and oleander made a wonderful backdrop for our seating under the lemon tree. Sunset marked the changeover from the warmth of the days to the modest fresh of the evenings. Cooled Costa Esmeralda or a ruby Marqués filled the glass; candles lit the tray with small cuts of pata negra, mancheco cheese, and olives invitingly placed on the table. We relaxed and enjoyed the romantic setting.

We loved to be pampered, but it was up to us to produce the treat. Dorthe and I had our unspoken end-of-day routine. Swiftly, we would go through the house and clean up a bit: beach towels on the drying rack, bicycles inside, and things cleared away for another day. A shaveand-shower later, we complimented each other for dressing up. We would review the events and detail our dinner plans. Spain gave us our life back. We were dependent on each other. We were not isolated, but we were on our own. For our interests, companionship, and social arrangements, we relied on each other. We were happy and in love. We were together 24-7 and occupied with life and the two of us. Still, there were not enough hours in a day; we never made it to bed before midnight. Turning in went with saying, "Thank you for a beautiful day." The bud of the hibiscus left on the night table would be fully open in the morning.

One day during the stay, my old friend and colleague, Javier, asked me over lunch in Puerto Banus if he could ask a very personal question: "Were you afraid of death?" I was not surprised by the question nor did it take me long to formulate the answer. I guess that I had contemplated the question one way or another since I had been hospitalized and had the ones I love at my bedside. "No, I am not afraid of death; I am afraid for the ones I love and leave behind."

In hindsight, I identified several key areas ranging from medical through mental to physical. Whatever way you define recovery, the first six months are gone before you know it. Once you are back on the learning track, there is no end to it. That is true for even the healthiest of people.

Several figures throughout the book illustrate the progress of my recovery. It is my attempt to answer questions that medical specialists could not easily commit to. My perception of total recovery over time has little objective meaning. Despite the lack of absolute value to the medical world, I believe that the illustrations and the accompanying text can help others with their own assessment.

The first graph represents the whole of the individual medical, mental, and physical key areas. I decided to present total recovery as the mathematical average of the sum of abilities and well-being prior to the brain stroke. The approach whereby all key areas are weighed equally is easily criticized. For one thing, it is difficult to identify all of the primary fields of recovery, and many are intertwined—such as balance and vision or handling stress and multitasking. To assign a level of significance, which changes over time, to each key area, further complicates an objective representation. Swallowing is a good example: it is a primary function in the early phase of recovery but, once mastered, the importance is rapidly surpassed by other functions that become apparent at a later stage.

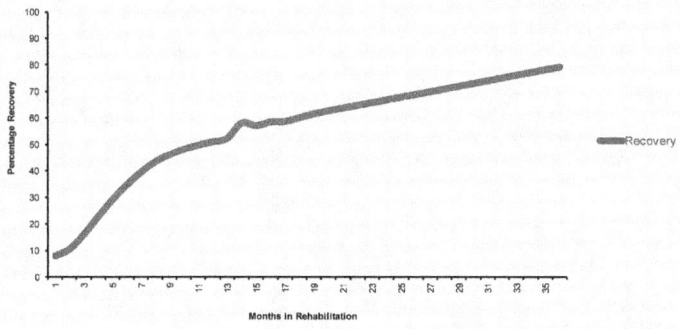

Figure 1. Total Recovery

Nevertheless, I feel comfortable with the progression of the curve overall. It does resemble my perception of recovery quite accurately. I may have rated my recovery slightly better during the first half of the rehabilitation period, but that might well be under the influence of my optimism. The progress of recovery flattens after that. By the end of the three-year period, I would indeed rate my recovery satisfactorily, but I must admit that is only true as long as I can command the expectations put upon me.

The other graphs in this book show the individual key areas that form the basis for the construction of the recovery curve as the average of functions. The key areas are divided into medical, mental, and physical. Swallowing, using the voice, and eyesight are deemed medical; whereas, balance, strength, and coordination are physical. Energy, stress handling, and multitasking are considered primarily mental. Throughout this book, each of the key areas is described in more detail within the framework of my personal experiences.

The Caregiver

"To have and to hold...from this day forward...for better, for worse...for richer, for poorer...in sickness or in health... to love and to cherish...'til death do us part." The marriage vows were inviolable to Dorthe. I was lucky that she took on the role of caregiver. Without her love and care, I would not be what I am today.

Support from the home front or a designated health-care professional is a necessity for an optimal recovery. The function of the patient's companion in rehabilitation is versatile. It is a partnership of give and take—not one or the other— mutual respect, and ultimate trust. The abstract qualities of the individual are applied to concrete areas such as communication and the additional care. Attending to the physical and emotional needs of the patient requires the virtues of an angel in disguise. The perfect candidate is probably somebody you would like to marry—if you have not already done so.

The generally accepted term to describe the role of the primary support person is "caregiver." If not a professional, usually a family member assumes the responsibility. Unexpectedly, the caregiver may stumble on what turns out to be a demanding job. The dependency of the patient on the caregiver can be much deeper, broader, and longer than initially anticipated.

Most hospitals employ a social counselor to discuss the expectations and fundamentals of this post. Among the personal characteristics of the caregiver are unselfishness, patience, and compassion. The involvement will test the pillars of their mental strength and stability. To share the emotions of the patient is not an easy task. Both caregiver and patient have their often-intertwined hopes, values, and dreams. Being that close effectively means defining one-another's mode of thought and mood. They become emotionally dependent. In that partnership, it is important to stimulate each other. Keep the relationship positive and motivating. One way is to share the pride of achieving milestones. Awards go to both.

The caregiver needs care too. Compassion and empathy create stress, which weighs heavily on his or her well-being. The experiences of the home front are often equally lonely and helpless. Looking after the caregiver commonly falls on friends and family. They should try to facilitate a break for the caregiver from time-to-time by taking over the role for a short period.

Care starts by preventing loneliness. That may be easier said than done. Travel time and distance might hinder frequent visits. The question becomes: "How long can the caregiver keep up with commuting?" The two rehabilitation hospitals where I stayed were located in the countryside. Incorporating detours between home and work was no longer possible. As my abilities increased, Dorthe's visits became less frequent.

Eventually, I was the one doing the traveling by bus and ferry to be home for the weekends. Both centers provided family members the opportunity to rent a room for the weekend. I met a fantastic positive elderly couple. They shared a room permanently. The husband, the caregiver, took part in all the exercises either actively or along the sideline. He was always by her side. Witnessing the kind-heartedness was touching. I can think of no better example of people who refused to be separated. Most of us mortals do not have that luxury, and we need to find more common ways to uphold our loyalty.

Not feeling misplaced or forgotten adds to the patient's spirits and self-esteem. Both of these are characteristics that are valuable in recovery. Simple things make hospital life more agreeable and personal: family pictures, a training outfit, music, books, and puzzles or other brainteasers. You do not need much in the hospital, but when you can surround yourself with a choice of things to do or wear, life is a lot more interesting. Understanding the patient's comfort zone provides some good hints about what he or she will appreciate.

News travels fast in the family and among friends. The overwhelming interest in my development and the sympathy I received were invaluable. On the other hand, Dorthe's ability to respond to the continuous stream of inquiries, however positive and welcome, was limited. Previous experiences had taught her that setting priorities was in order. Happily, her direct contacts offered to off-load her by informing others.

Internal communication focused on the nurses, specialists, and therapists. Initially, it was aimed at providing information about my personality and preferences. That was the easy part. Receiving information is more difficult, particularly if one is untrained for the job and jargon. Dorthe got a crash course in the system's lingo and the way health care works. She sought involvement by asking open questions and offering assistance. It required a lot of careful listening to understand what was actually being said. There was room for trust and confidence but not for assumptions and misunderstandings.

Much of the communication in the hospital relates to care and cure. There are medical updates— possible complications, examinations, and treatments to discuss—and the daily information exchanges with the nurses. Dorte communicated on my behalf, substituted my rasping voice, and complemented my marginal brainpower. Patiently, she would give me a popular version of the medical ins-and-outs and unfold plans and purposes. My trust in her was unconditional. Skillfully, she managed to maintain my sense of active participation without lessening my fragile self-esteem.

If anybody knows what is happening on the hospital floor it is the nurses. They pass on their findings from shift to shift. You can always get ahold of them when visiting and bombard them with your questions. As a volunteer, the caregiver complements their work. A good relationship with the staff is the beginning of a win-win situation. Dorthe would ask about their observations, medical opinions, information on nutrition and medication, or how to best prepare for my homecoming during the weekends. She practiced under their supervision. Being included and relied on by the staff increased her competence.

Coming home in a wheelchair for a weekend leave required a great deal of groundwork. Furniture had to be re-arranged to create easy access to the bathroom and bedroom. However, the preparation goes beyond removing obstacles. Get ahold of the name and number of the contact at the hospital so that in case of an emergency, help is only a call away. Needs, medication, and nutrition must be well understood and, in my case, how to feed directly into the stomach had to be practiced in advance. An assisted living situation at home may require the use of special techniques when it comes to lifting or holding up a person. Only partially capable of self-care, I needed help to shower and dress. It all fell on on Dorthe.

My recovery progressed steadily. We went out whenever the weather allowed: at first with the wheelchair, later on foot with a stick, and eventually hand in hand. It was Dorthe's turn to be spoiled. In the relaxed atmosphere of a fancy restaurant downtown, we dwelt on our future and made plans. Daydreaming and exploring imaginary horizons is a gift reserved for humans; we enjoyed it.

It was not always easy on her when people thought I was tipsy. My poor balance easily created that misunderstanding. At times, I wished I had a walking cane to accentuate my condition. Bluntly, Dorthe rejected the idea. She preferred a subtle comment or obvious gesture—just clear enough for people to understand that my sway was more of a handicap than the effect of alcohol. Avoiding false impressions became second nature.

Find Satisfaction In Rehabilitation

We are all unique. All things being equal, the perception differs and reactions vary. Our rational and emotional response to a change in situation is the product of a lifetime of accumulated knowledge, skill, and sensations. This time around, the change is within us. Suddenly our capacity, capability, and behavior are affected by an aggregate of biological and psychological factors.

The effect from a brain stroke differs from mild to grave depending on the type of stroke and the permanent damage done. Unprepared, we find ourselves in a hospital and moved to a rehabilitation center or nursing home.

I have been lucky enough to live through the shock of being fully incapacitated, arriving at a new and rewarding life, and having the opportunity to share my experiences with others. There is no single recipe to successful recovery. The causes, effects and reactions differ too much. Nevertheless, there are common denominators in the recovery process that are worth mentioning. In whole or in part, the following synopsis can help people to get more satisfaction out of their job of rehabilitation.

Look forward and think positive. Rehabilitation is a job that cannot be delegated. As soon as you realize that things do not get better unless you work for it—and that does not take very long—you take on the job of physical and mental reconditioning.

Once begun, life is not about what you have lost but about what you have gained. That very moment you have marked a reference point for your achievements during rehabilitation. Taking pride in renewed capabilities is a strong motivator, particularly if you add a twist of self-competiveness to it.

There is no room for negative thoughts or people that openly pity you and undermine your self-esteem. Dismiss a person, maybe another patient, who drags you back in time by reminding you of his or your own capabilities in bygone days. These thoughts are not constructive. Once in recovery, whatever the scope or acceleration, only progress matters. To maintain and protect a positive attitude, one has to be realistic and pick the battles with care. Pick those fights that you know that you can win, and give yourself enough time to win them.

Balance the use of energy. It is common for people that have suffered from a stroke to enjoy a siesta and a short nap before or after their evening meal—and not just for the pleasure of it. The brain is working hard to process the day's impressions and actions. Functioning deteriorates when you are tired. Without a regular break, you will most likely run out of steam before the day is over. Rest well before you are drained from energy, drink enough water or fruit juice, and eat sugars to speed up recuperation.

Balancing the use of energy is something one must learn to master. It requires getting to know how large your reserves are and what your rate of energy consumption is. Combined with forward planning, it helps you to get most out of the day. Top-off your batteries before a nice evening with friends, exercising, shopping, enjoying a hobby, or working. Once you come to grips with properly anticipating the quantity of energy needed, it creates extra room to be active.

By now, my friends and family know about my addiction to the siesta and I do not have to apologize any longer for temporarily withdrawing from the crowd.

Communicate. Talk to people so that they can talk back. Appreciate the pep talks, compliments, and well-meant concerns you get in response. An open attitude toward communication reduces the possibility of social isolation. Welcome people who address you directly. Personal contact creates understanding. In turn, it distributes the load that you are carrying.

Communication can be in writing too. I use short quarterly newsletters to keep distant friends and relatives informed about our well-being and our future plans. Focus on what's right, not on what's wrong. People enjoy a positive dialogue, not a litany of complaints.

The power of humor cannot be overestimated. Humor and self-mockery can tone down the gravity of the situation and create room to discuss a serious topic in a relaxed and constructive fashion.

Work for it. You can pray for a miracle, but rehabilitation is a do-it-yourself job. In recovery, accept all the help you can get from above, specialists, friends, and family. But the bottom line is that it cannot be outsourced. Only personal devotion will yield results. You must be willing to match ambition with commitment.

Rehabilitation is physically demanding. Mentally, the journey is full of contrasting emotions (joy and sadness), high spirits, and demoralizing experiences. Goals can be out of your league or they may take longer to achieve than predicted; whatever the reason, always deliver to the best of your ability. You cannot cut corners. Do not be beaten by the track; rather try another route instead.

Accept compliments for what they are. At home, we have always called it the "Oh and Ah" factor. Nobody can do without it. It does not take much to pause what you are doing and divert positive attention to somebody who is working hard to achieve something.

Perhaps your recipient is the sweet old lady down the street who is nursing the rose bushes in her front garden. After you have delivered her your "Ohs and Ahs," she will most likely get even sweeter, and her roses will blossom as never before. Your attention motivates her.

The trick is learning to accept compliments for what they are. Compliments are a motivator to carry on despite the seeming loneliness in which something is carried out. The same is true for the obvious pep talk. Do not reject it because you think you can see through it, but accept it because in the bottom of your heart you know you need it. Use it to your advantage.

Train your brain. To overcome back pain, you follow a prescribed training program. What do you do if you have a problem with the brain?

Spending time in the hospital makes your brain lazy. All the thinking is done for you. However, this is not the time for a vacation. Most likely your comprehension is slow, you're easily stressed, you have a short span of concentration, and doing just one thing at a time is enough to wear you out. As soon as your condition allows for it, try to spend a few minutes per day on a workout of the brain, and build it up slowly. Do this along with your physical or medical treatments.

Make sure that brainteasers are varied and enjoyable. Just like fitness training, a brain workout can actually help you to relax. When you are up to it, consider drawing or modeling clay. Not all brain training has to be logical, and it is good for your fine-motor coordination too.

Keep up your self-esteem. It is easy to forget about your behavior, dignity, and appearance. After a few days in the hospital, you start to realize the severity of the situation, and your self-esteem might hit a low. Now is a good time for a boost. It is probably more important than ever as you contemplate what lies ahead.

Initially, you spend most of the time in bed. Unless you do something about it, you will not feel any smarter. Call on the help of nurses and family. It starts with fresh pajamas, a shave, and a haircut when due.

The way you look will rub off on the way you feel. Self-esteem is the overall evaluation and appraisal of your own worth. It is reflected in your attitude and appearance; it is a characteristic of your personality. Be true to yourself but appreciate that the qualities of an individual are unknown to the people you have become acquainted with in the hospital; to the staff and fellow patients you are a stranger at first.

Compromising with that reality may contribute to a harmonious environment from which you will certainly benefit.

Be aware of the danger of apathy when socially isolated during recovery. A long stay in rehabilitation can make you indifferent and insensitive toward others. On the other hand, a change of surroundings, a gathering, or an outing inspires involvement and enthusiasm. Most centers offer an activity program. Do not say, "No" too hastily when invited to participate. There is a good reason someone asked you.

"Being competent to cope with the challenges of life, and being worthy of happiness." This is a little broader definition, but the double twist fits the demands of *Reconditioning Mind and Body for a New and Rewarding Lifestyle* perfectly. Show your commitment to successful recovery and demonstrate your willpower. The self-confidence will fuel your drive, create respect, and deem you worthy of happiness.

Be a good patient. The two main elements are: not to take personal care for granted and to realize that what good you give reflects upon you. It is not easy to find yourself suddenly in a hospital among professionals. They are trained for the job. But how about the patient?

I assume that you are used to saying, "please," "thank you," and "good morning." Those few words—combined with patience and a smile—will get you a long way. It is empathy working both ways. Be social and offer assistance. Simple things, like clearing away your plate after dinner or tidying up your training equipment, are good exercises too.

Professionalism, along with correct medical decisions, is something you may rightfully demand, but building a good working relationship with the hospital staff is very much up to the patient and caregiver. You may find yourself turned over to nurses and physiotherapists for months, so why not try to make the best out of it? Just like the patient, every professional is human too. They are not your personal servants. The patient's behavior should reflect that understanding.

Define your goals and objectives. Setting meaningful objectives is something that most people do not master very well. The reason is that goals and objectives set outside of their context are doomed to fail, or the desire to achieve evaporates over time. A long time ago, I learned about the SMART rule. SMART stands for Specific, Measurable, Achievable, Realistic, and Timed. Consider each of these components before committing yourself to something.

Be aware of the fact that trying to master something that is unrealistic or cannot be achieved within the time frame you have given yourself will frustrate your motivation. Frustration comes from the drive to change things that are out of reach. With that understanding, there is no aggravation and consequently less stress.

In general, small steps are easier to accomplish, so do not try to run before you can walk. My advice is to break down your tasks to manageable chunks for the short and medium term.

Be proud of your achievements. Look for elements of self-motivation in every bit of progress you make. Commemorate your achievements. Nothing gives a greater satisfaction than breaking a record, mastering something new, or showing off your latest achievements. The journey of rehabilitation is made in many small steps, each a stepping-stone toward a new and rewarding lifestyle.

Swallowing

My appetite was unchanged. One thing was a mystery: my sudden, inexplicable taste for chocolate and sweets. The variety of new flavors was irresistible and longed-for more than ever.

After the stroke, I could not taste or swallow. A lack of reflexes blocked any intake. Under normal circumstances, swallowing is the result of perfect teamwork of the tongue and throat and contractions of the digestive track. It is up to the brain stem to invoke the function. A domino effect of involuntary actions and reactions is the result; breathing and speech is temporarily barred by closing the windpipe and folding the vocal cords. The control program had been erased by the crash of the brain stem's little super computer. With exercise, the therapist tried to retrieve the function from the back-up that resided somewhere in the brain. The body is an intelligent piece of engineering. Would the system be smart enough to recognize the repetitive stimulus and react accordingly?

Deliberately invoking the muscle reactions to move food from mouth to stomach is hard, if not impossible. Trying against all odds is tricky as there is the risk of choking. Swallowing is taken for granted—up to the point where you abruptly lose the ability. The impact is far reaching. Obviously, it means no eating or drinking. Medication and saliva can no longer go the trusted route. Any intake through the mouth just ends. The result is a life without taste.

Consequently, feeding goes the intravenous route. Eventually, the infusions clog up and the nurse has to find a new spot in the vein. In my case, direct infusion in the artery extended the input of fluid but increased the risk of an infection. As I grew weaker, my resistance went down rapidly, and the last thing the doctors needed was an infection of the blood or arteries or the possibility of pneumonia. The latter had been a realistic threat for some time. There was a real danger of food or water getting into the lungs. Normally, the flap under the tongue and tightening of the vocal cords block the top of the windpipe during swallowing. However, my tongue muscles were weak, and one of the vocal cords was paralyzed. The usefulness of both intravenous options was soon running out. They could only provide a solution for a few weeks at best. Trying a long-term solution, the peg, was forthcoming. The peg is a simple piece of plumbing that goes directly through the wall of the stomach with a small tube to which you can connect an oversized syringe.

My stomach did not welcome the daily measure of liquid food with the direct feed and went on strike time-after-time. It was cause for worry. I was losing weight quickly, and I became weaker and more vulnerable by the day. The biggest problem was the intake of water. We produce over a liter of saliva per day. Being unable to swallow your saliva creates an immediate problem. Instead of recycling, I had to spit it out. Dehydration was in the danger zone, my blood pressure was sinking, and my stomach did not accept food. After putting me on red alert, the nurses carefully measured and recorded everything that went in and out.

My biggest nightmare was the hiccups. There are dozens of potential causes: some are trivial; others, highly complex. Directly or indirectly, some relate to the nervous system or a deficiency in the brain stem. From time to time, the nasty reaction played up. Whenever the dose of liquid high-nutrition food was too aggressive, it triggered the spasmodic contraction of the diaphragm. Stopping the feed and slowly rebuilding the intake from scratch was the only way to stop the reflex. The boys counted my hiccups and did some quick arithmetic—up to hundreds of times per hour. It could last for days only to go away once I fell asleep from exhaustion. The experience was exhausting, and it caused setbacks in my nutrition.

The doctor tried medication to calm down my stomach to end the hiccups. The drug made me throw up. I panicked of near drowning. I was fuming when the nurse commented on the quality of the drug. It could not have been the intention to cure me from the hiccups with an old home remedy of scaring me to death. For the moment, I had lost my sense of humor; the next day I had pneumonia. How to suppress the hiccups effectively remains a mystery. Biologists suggest that the reflex is an evolutionary remnant of amphibian breathing. I would have been happy to play the frog if the doctors could have found me a princess to break the spell.

We have the ability to consciously command many of our biological systems. There is a sense of control over the function. Swallowing falls in a different category. The ability is controlled by the subconscious. It was a matter of endless trials to stimulate a reaction. After I spent weeks sipping thickened water and hundreds of tiny spoons of thinned porridge, the therapist successfully managed to reanimate the throat movements and contractions of the digestive track. From then on, progress accelerated.

I enjoyed the taste of food. Finishing a small bowl required concentration; an hour would easily pass by. Under strict supervision, I trained the brain and muscles to work the food down. Alert as the overseer was for any mishap, there was no room for talking: trial and no error. "One thing at a time" was the credo. It took several months to eat enough to increase the calorie intake to a level where it could replace the artificial feeding. I gained weight, strength, and energy. When I moved on to the specialized rehabilitation hospital, I was eating a real breakfast, lunch, and dinner in the lounge together with some of the other patients. By then I was patient off—at least, medically speaking.

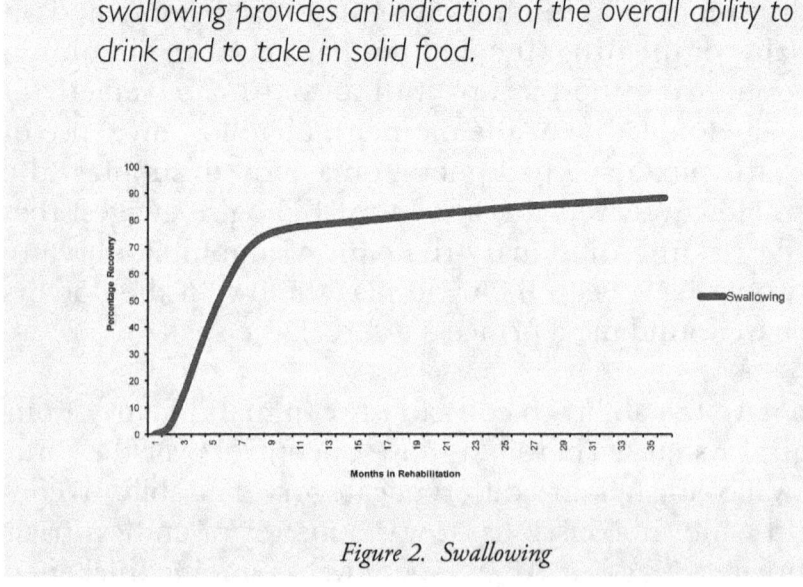

In the context of rehabilitation, my definition of swallowing provides an indication of the overall ability to drink and to take in solid food.

Figure 2. Swallowing

Rating the ability to swallow directly after the stroke was straightforward: zero percent. Of all my disabilities, it had the biggest impact on my well-being. The effects were instantaneous. I lived on the edge of dehydration— far below the normal calorie intake—lost weight and energy, and encountered medical complications. It took several months before I was able to drink and eat a little. Slowly, the function returned. From that point onward, the progression was steep and stayed on the upswing for approximately half a year. I regained weight and felt the positive effects on my strength and energy. Within a year, approximately eighty percent of the function recovered. After that, the pace of improvement lessened.

Today, I rate the ability just under ninety percent, which is absolutely acceptable. I eat almost everything. Only a few inconveniences remain. Eating and drinking need concentration. Knocking back a glass in big gulps is out of the question. It is best to steer clear of a blend of soft and hard ingredients or even a crispy snack. Talking over dinner calls for a deliberate pause; otherwise, I start coughing. There is also the need to sit up. When in bed, swallowing my saliva is still difficult. The contractions of the gullet and movements of the tongue are weaker than they used to be.

There are pros and cons to everything. I am not tempted to talk with my mouth full, and I get the opportunity to really taste what I eat and drink.

Energy Balance

Without energy, there is no existence. Practically, human existence implies activity—at least an active brain. Activity costs energy; make sure that you always have enough. When you maintain a healthy energy balance, you get a wealth of pleasure from participating, giving, receiving, or sharing. A social get-together can be most satisfying as long as you have the energy to bring into play.

A way of looking at the available energy, irrespective of capability or capacity, is considering the time one is awake and can move about. In my case, a surplus of energy was probably one of the least pressing things to quantify. Initially, I had hardly enough to meet the demand of a single hour. The mind absorbed every bit; not a single move or swallow was without awareness. Every action, however small, was discrete, mentally rehearsed, and executed with painstaking concentration.

Given the amount of energy it takes to recuperate from a stroke, it is not surprising that initially most of the time is spend resting in a hospital bed. My presence in intensive care was only physical. The weeks after being in intensive care, I slept away most of the day. The unconscious had made restoring my biological stability and life support systems a priority. The neurological disarray influenced the energy consumption more than my physical state. Interruptions by the scheduled hospital routines and short visits by family were enough to wear me out.

For months, I lived on a supply of high-protein liquid pumped directly into my stomach. It provided limited fuel, had no taste, and was far from an elegant way of dining; I lost a fifth of my body weight. Muscles deteriorate surprisingly fast when you are short on nutrition and restricted to your bed. When the ability to swallow returned, my energy increased steeply. The acceleration in upturn was revitalizing as the intake of calories took effect. The therapeutically motivated exercises that followed improved my mental and physical condition simultaneously. They had a positive impact on my capability to uphold my energy level. Within a year, the pounds returned, but they were not distributed as nicely as I would have liked. A lesser quantity would have saved me a lot of fat-burning and body-toning exercises afterward.

Balancing the use of energy is essential. You need to know when to stop and stock up your reserve; I learned it the hard way. At first, I overestimated my potential and did not hold back on my exercises. As a result, my nonstop drive to rehabilitate started to burn up my reserve. Therapists had warned me of the negative effects of pushing my training beyond its limits. Ignoring their advice—my determination to recover was matched by my stubbornness—it proved to be too much indeed. Without energy contingency, I would, figuratively speaking, cave in within less than an hour. Recharging a completely dead battery takes dreadfully long; up to several days is no exception. To top-off well before running on fumes takes only a short time; like in youthful days, a power nap may be sufficient to continue.

A loss of energy would lead to a diminishing concentration and difficulties with my eyesight and balance. In turn, that would make me feel ungainly and insecure and would quickly result in irritation with others and myself; for other people I would be a grumpy nuisance. This is not a nice situation to be in for either yourself or the folks around you, so avoid it if possible. The correct energy balance is maintained best by anticipating future plans and taking your rest well before events. Nowadays, I take an afternoon break and a power nap before or after dinner to ensure that I have enough energy in reserve to enjoy the evening. I would not blame the respite at midday solely on the stroke. Age is another factor, and when in Spain, I had grown accustomed to their legendary siesta.

The need for a regular rest does not stop me from spending full days with friends or travel. With a bit of creativity, it is not difficult to find a place for your short retreat. When it is time for a pause, there is always a corner on the sofa to withdraw for a power nap. When on the road, why not try a picnic spot, the grass in the park, or a beach chair? In a busy city, even a solarium will do; you will love the sense of freedom. I have always been very proper, but now my uncomplicated choice of the when and where for my time-out adds to my independence. Keeping up appearances is to nobody's benefit.

The sun, vitamins, and the siesta had a healthy effect on my energy. Dorthe and I got on our mountain bikes every day. What had been a frightening experience at first, turned out to be our favorite outdoor activity. We loved a trip along the Spanish beaches via the Paseo Maritimo or to our local fitness center in Puerto Banus. On the bike, I found it easier to maintain my balance than by foot; speed must have something to do with it. A healthy respect of Spanish drivers for cyclists is something I fortunately quickly developed. Motorists carefully avoid eye contact not to lose a presumed right of way. I quickly learned when to use the sidewalk and zebra crossings to navigate through town.

When the energy reserve remains untouched, you are not limited by quantity but by distribution. Ad hoc changes to my timetable proved destructive. Activity planning and the communication of my plans was a good way to solicit consideration by my environment. Stretching my capabilities too far undermined the attention level first; next came the negative side effects: silly mistakes, bad decisions, sloppy communication, and a poor control of emotions.

I avoid drastic changes to the plans for the day. Suppose that in the morning we agreed to go shopping or join a workout class in the late afternoon. To suddenly move that forward a couple of hours would mean that I would have to put off my siesta. Going through with a change of plans, will unwittingly, but likely, spoil the fun of the trip to town or ruin my fitness training. The people around me know that I need my afternoon rest to make it happily through the day. It is not a lack of flexibility which makes the original plan seem carved in stone; the ability to accept change is restricted by the priority of maintaining a healthy energy balance. The better I plan on the short and medium term, the easier it is to anticipate the use of energy and to keep going.

In the context of rehabilitation, my definition of energy provides an indication of the time available to be active.

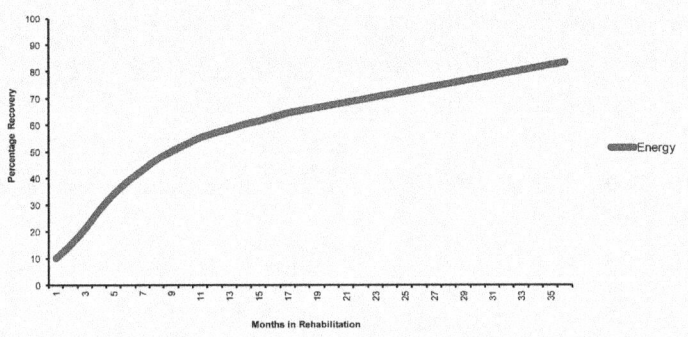

Figure 3. Energy

The energy chart shows my progression over the three years following the brain stroke. It presents an observation that could be meaningful to other patients or create for family and friends a better understanding of the condition. It could assist in setting expectations for recovery.

During the first month in the hospital, I would not dare to value my energy level higher than needed to undergo the pampering of the nurses and to be aware of visitors. It took months to regain approximately one-third of my old level. The curve is the steepest in the beginning, which I attribute largely to my renewed ability to swallow and the start of my rehabilitation program. Halfway through the observed period, I estimate my energy at two-thirds. The speed of recovery flattened after that. At the end of the three-year period, I rate it as acceptable.

Nowadays, much of my focus is on brain training in parallel with conditioning of the physique; both are large energy consumers. Whatever the progress, I should benefit from the healthy lifestyle, but I expect to continue making improvements at the same rate, or slightly less, as over the past year. It will probably take a little while before I will be nearing full recovery…but who's counting? At worst, my current energy limitation is merely an inconvenience, not a handicap. Interestingly enough, I found that you quickly fall back once you stop exercising. To keep the overall level of recovery stable, you are doomed to keep it up.

Voice

As children, we used to blow air between the two sides of a folded leaf to get a high shrieking tone: the tighter the fold, the higher the pitch. It springs to mind whenever I envision how our vocal cords work.

The characteristic of your voice is a unique attribute; it is part of your personality. The tone, timbre, pitch, and volume are all part of who you are: "Hello, it's you. I recognize your voice." Your voice is like a fingerprint. Losing your voice is like losing your identity; you also lose self-confidence.

The sounds you make when talking or singing, and the emotions given thereby, are the result of more than the work put in by the vocal cords. Your physical build and muscles influence the characteristics. The lungs produce the airflow, with sufficient pressure, to set off the vibration. The cords are flat triangular bands—like a curtain at the top of the windpipe. They start to flutter in the wind. The tighter the curtains are drawn, the higher the sound. The voice box in your throat adjusts tone and pitch by varying the tension of the vocal cords. Fine-tuning is done by articulation with the tongue, palate, and muscles in the cheek and lips.

The voice system is very sophisticated, and the interaction with the brain function for speech makes it a beautiful instrument. However, whatever way you look at it, the functioning of the vocal cords is fundamental. Trying to manipulate your voice is useless unless the vocal cords produce the basic sound.

In my case, one cord was paralyzed and had dropped to the side. The gap had doubled in size. The other now worked for two. My speech was soft and had lost intonation. Talking made me tired as I spilled air on sounds that were difficult to identify. We jokingly referred to my new image as that of Don Corleone, the hoarse-spoken Mafioso stereotype in *The Godfather*. Sexy or not, it was a frustrating experience. Losing your voice complicates daily life; socializing or any other verbal contact becomes extremely cumbersome. For me, making phone calls was out of the question.

Uncontrolled intonation paved the way for misunderstandings. Often, it is not what you say, but how you say it. Simple sayings can be perceived very differently from how they were intended. It is easy to place the emphasis on the wrong word or syllable. Friendly curiosity can come across as aggressive judgment. There is a big difference between "What are you doing?" and "What are you doing!" Without intonation, it is hard to put emotion in the voice. Saying things with a smile becomes solely dependent on one's facial expression. Watching your body language is suddenly critical. This may be difficult, as a stroke may affect your posture. People may think that a stroke led to a change in character. That is not necessarily true. The cause may be much more down to earth. Learning how to avoid misconception due to the

limited ability of the voice takes a lot of apologies and training. The speech therapist plays a crucial role in the latter.

Borgny, the therapist at the Sunnaas Rehabilitation hospital, took me on as her patient in speech therapy and continued mending my swallowing disorder. It is common that the
same specialist attends both; structure, muscles, and nerves
overlap. We practiced daily. Many of the exercises were obvious in nature once we understood the problem. With a model
of the anatomy at hand, she pointed out how the various functions worked. The visualization helped my mind to focus on
the specific purpose of the exercises. In her practice, she used
a whole repertoire: it started with making grimaces to loosen
up the facial muscles and was followed by a few deep yawns.

Air is spilled when the vocal cords do not touch. Halfway
through a sentence, I would run out of breath. Speaking was
very tiresome. One of the first things the speech therapist
focused on was my breathing and regulating the flow and pressure. For the training, she used a simple tool: a plastic bottle
filled with a few inches of water and a plastic tube for a straw.
I practiced my breathing with the diaphragm rather than the
chest: take a deep breath and exhale, for as long as possible,
through the tube. The stream of bubbles showed the quality of
the airflow; her stopwatch recorded the time. At first, I felt quite
silly—an adult blowing bubbles. Then, Borgny mirrored every
assignment. It was a clever approach. By sharing my embarrass-
ment, she kept me motivated; she even created some form of
competition. Despite the laughs, she kept a serious undertone.
Progress was slow, but the effects were definitely noticeable.
'Slow' meant measured in weeks rather than days.

The results of the therapy became particularly noticeable
when reading aloud. Reading children's books was fun. In

general, the sentences are short and simple but a challenge when it comes to intonation. Nursery rhymes proved to be a good way to practice the pitch of the voice. The octave '*do-re-mi-fa-sol-la-ti-do*' was a tough one. Even from a low bass, I never managed to reach the upper end of the musical scale. Those high tones were beyond my reach. Playing the old tape recordings gave evidence of my advancement. Sentences became longer, intonation and volume improved, and the gasps for air were less noticeable.

The specialist had diagnosed vocal paresis with a fiber-optic scope. Although he could confirm the cause of the problem visually, he was hesitant to operate. This particular paralysis may heal itself spontaneously. He wanted to wait a year before carrying out surgery.

One of two techniques is commonly practiced. One method narrows the gap; the other improves the contact surface. The surgeon chose the first and pushed the paralyzed cord permanently in the mid position. The intervention was uncomplicated; it took precision and a small pin through the outer wall of the voice box. Nothing but a small scar shows. The second method thickens the edge of the vocal cord—temporarily by injecting small amounts of fat, or permanently with molded silicone implants. I keep that option in reserve.

A vocal cord placed in the mid position reduces the passage of air. This is a consideration for the surgeon. Since the operation, I have been working hard on my physical condition. Contrary to thought, I have not experienced any limitations in my air intake other than what I would contribute to being out of shape. I have not felt short of breath. Nevertheless, there is no talking while sporting.

The swelling after the operation created a laughable side effect. My voice was difficult to control. Unexpectedly, I would shock myself, and others, with a sudden step up in pitch. Within a few weeks, the effect disappeared, but overall, the improvement lasted. Excitedly, I surprised my friends with a phone call. To get the most out of my renewed speech ability, I continued therapy. A few months later, improvements were only marginal, and I decided to focus on my Spanish.

In the context of rehabilitation, my definition of voice provides an indication of the quality of volume, clarity, pitch, and intonation of speech.

The speech ability had almost fully disappeared immediately after the stroke. Actually, what remained became slightly worse during the first month. This was probably due to fatigue of the vocal cord that still worked, or it may have taken time before the paralyzed cord fully parted in the open position and its thickness shrank. The year thereafter, the quality of the voice improved significantly. This is solely attributed to the skilled therapists. Thanks to them, I almost doubled my quality of speech. At the time of surgery, I had rebuilt my ability to roughly one-third. I could make myself understood in face-to-face situations. Making phone calls was not possible.

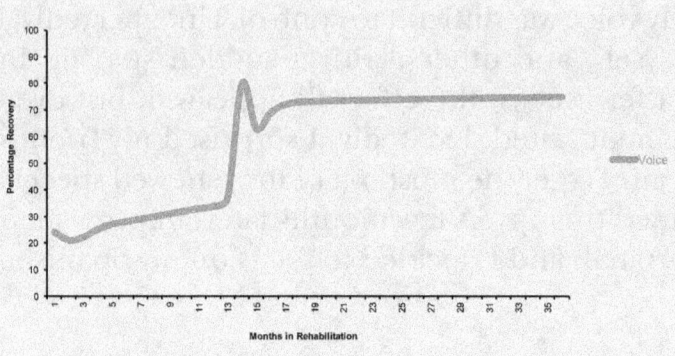

Figure 4. Voice

The operation during which the surgeon permanently placed the paralyzed vocal cord in the mid position was a big success. The sudden peak in the curve depicts it. My ability to speak doubled instantaneously. It slightly dropped thereafter as the swelling, caused by the operation, disappeared. Approximately two-thirds of the full ability remained.

Additional training was required to learn how to best control my renewed ability. Six months after the operation, further progress was hardly noticeable, and the therapy discontinued.

Today, there is still ample room for improvement. My voice does not carry very far. However, I can get by in most normal situations but find it difficult to speak in a noisy environment, when in a large crowd, or if stressed. For social purposes, I can make short phone calls. Looking at it from the bright side, I have become a much better listener.

Vision

The eyes and the brain form an integrated system. Seeing starts when the eye focuses on its surroundings and projects the image onto a light-sensitive membrane (the retina) in the back of the eye. The retina serves as a transducer for the conversion of the picture to neuronal signals. The brain interprets, draws conclusions, and lets the body know if it thinks that it is worth responding.

After the stroke, I saw everything double. It distorted my surroundings. Normally, both eyes focus on the same point in the distance. A slight offset at the base, determined by the spacing between the eyes, gives you the ability to measure depth. When you see double, one eye looks at an object while the line of sight of the other is slightly off and focuses differently. This results in seeing the same object twice at a slightly different position. This form of squinting is not just disturbing when looking at a single object, but it has an effect on the boundary lines of the ceiling, walls, and floor or the position of letters across the page of a book. You can imagine the negative effect on your balance.

Vision and balance are obviously related. My poor eyesight hampered my stability. Then again, blind people can have very good balance. The permanent damage to their vision is compensated by an increased sensitivity to change. In my case, the additional signals—for instance from the inner ear or touch—were just as defective. My control center had the almost impossible task of solving the equilibrium equation.

Expert support awaited on the peninsula of Nesodden. Karin, the therapist who specialized in eyesight at Sunnaas Rehabilitation Hospital, was from the old school. She was German, pragmatic, and thorough. To my surprise, her office was not stuffed with a bank of optical and electronic equipment. Instead, her practically furnished room with a beautiful view over the Oslo fjord was sparsely equipped with relatively simple tools, study books, and prisms. It matched her approach to diagnostics and problem solving. It was more the library of a professor than a clinical laboratory of an optician.

With ease, Karin diagnosed the core of the problem: the movement of my right eye was not synchronized with the fixation of the left. She found no permanent damage to the eye or vision, which meant that, with exercise or special glasses, I would most likely be able to see properly again.

Karin came up with an utterly simple tool: she placed a long and narrow piece of cardboard with some markings on her desk and explained how to use it. It closely resembled a ruler of about a foot long with a small number of big black dots equally spaced along a line that ran in the middle from end to end. I had to place the artwork in front of my nose and focus hard on the dot at the far end of the line. At first, I saw two lines that crossed in space. The same dot that I was trying to get a fix on was hovering at the end of each of the two lines. Slowly, my eyes managed to force the dots on top of each other. Once I had managed to see one point only, I had to move my fixation closer and closer. The two lines started to cross on the dot. She was making me squint on purpose to undo the misalignment of the eye; to me she was a genius with her homemade 'gizmo.'

Training of the eye was entertaining. Within a few weeks, I played the dots like an octave on an instrument. A couple of times per day I did my exercise. I had been living in a cubist world. Slowly, the geometric deformations disappeared. My ability to read returned; characters found their place and formed words and numbers. My finger still had to track the sentences in order not to lose their position on the page, but I no longer needed to cover one eye to enjoy this restored dimension. I was overly happy with the progress and it worked its way into my motivation, balance, self-confidence, and more.

One Monday morning she gave me a present; I laughed, because it looked like a long pearl necklace. What was she thinking? Valentine's Day had passed. Big colorful pearls placed at knotted intervals formed a string of a few yards. Small loops at the end of the thin cord completed her design. She placed one of the loops over the door handle and asked me to hold the other under my nose and keep the line tight. It became apparent where she was headed with this. I had outgrown the small piece of cardboard, and it was time to extend my horizon.

Nowadays, the industry is so focused on technology that people tend to overlook the obvious and dismiss simple solutions in favor of complexity. Not Karin. Within a few months, she had eradicated my double vision with a cost-effective, practical tool; mixed with humor, patience, and play, she had done wonders. The result worked its way into all aspects of my rehabilitation. I was doing better and better, and by undertaking more and more, my recovery accelerated.

Peripheral vision is very inaccurate when it comes to high-definition imaging. What we see in the corner of the eye does not have to be very complete or exact. The primary function is to alert us of potential dangers and help us to quickly recognize familiar arrangements or changes in the background—not detailed visual examination. We can ignore the need for further inspection—as we do when walking past a fence—but as soon we record change, we are alert; the hint of a shadow approaching could be a nasty dog. This is similar to what happens when we follow the arrival signs at the airport and react immediately to an irregular movement in the crowd. The person waving in the background could be the one who is there to meet us. A sudden alteration in our field of vision draws the immediate attention. It triggers eye movement to place the blurred event in the center of our view while it focuses. The brain uses different areas to process information from the peripheral field than it does to evaluate input from our central vision. Parts of the brain that take care of what is happening in the peripheral field generate a fast reaction. Those areas seem to have developed a taste for processing large quantities of raw data rather than the quality of detail.

To examine what attracted my attention from the corner of the eye, I had to turn my head, find the object, and focus; each action was a discrete step. My poor balance complicated it. In practice, I was forced to stop walking and regain my balance before I could turn. Afraid to be visually distracted, I had the tendency to concentrate on what already lay within the straight line of sight. It was a simple priority: best image quality first.

My peripheral vision was tested by staring at the center of a hollow half-sphere while light points were projected randomly on the inside of the shell. Measuring the quality of the response whenever a point came into view generated a map of the field of vision for each eye. The edges of the map turned out a bit ragged but within the norm. There was no evidence of tunnel vision or damage. Additional tests, like those used for car drivers, revealed that my inability to respond quickly to what was happening in my wider surroundings boiled down to a slow reaction, which in turn was influenced by several factors: comprehension, a sluggish eye movement, and inadequate focus. With active training, I got rid of my double vision, but Karin could not help me any further. Training of the more refined muscles to enhance eye movement and speed of focus is continuous during everyday life. Overcoming those two limitations would require passive healing over time.

Comprehending what you see takes more than a gaze. The brain has to interpret the image in its context before it can respond. That function of cognitive recognition is usually incredibly fast, and so is the reaction in thought or action. For rehabilitation rather than linguistic purposes, I define comprehension as understanding what you see, or experience, by linking it to knowledge—but within an acceptable response time. Introducing the time factor underlines the need for speed. A split-second response is normal. After the stroke, my level of comprehension was low. The brain seemed to lack the processing power to construe input fast enough. Eventually, I would come to the right conclusion, but it could take a full second...sometimes even longer. In this condition, driving was out of the question. I was insecure; I did not dare to trust my vision at first sight nor my interpretation and actions. I double-checked all of my intentions. I would have to work on this. The mental feedback of my vision was not good enough in demanding situations. I decided to focus on what I could influence; I started training my brain.

In the context of rehabilitation, my definition of vision provides an indication of the quality of eyesight. It is expressed as a percentage of the vision prior to the brain stroke. The graph reflects the quality, irrespective of the need for glasses or renewal of prescription.

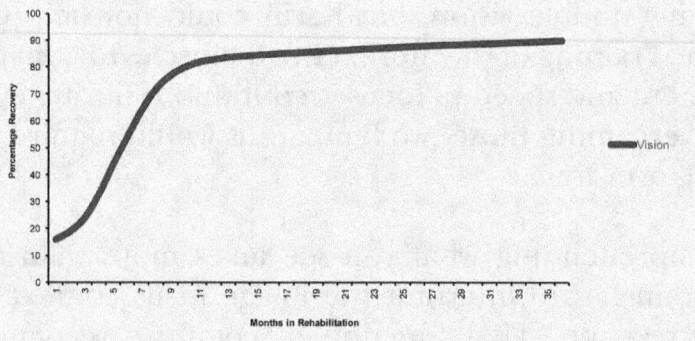

Figure 5. Quality of Vision

My eyesight after the stroke was marginal. The first and foremost problem was one of excessive double vision. My surroundings appeared badly deformed. It influenced my balance negatively, and reading was impossible. An eye patch offered some relief but prevented estimating depth. Permanently wearing an eye patch hampers recovery. Over time, the double vision lessened but not sensationally until I started with active eye training. It restored my central vision. Two-thirds of my vision returned within six months.

A year after the stroke, my vision had recovered almost entirely. I believe that this is due to a further self-teaching by the eye and brain in day-to-day life. The effects were particularly noticeable in the area of peripheral vision, improved eye movement, and better focusing. The last two years, progress has been slow but steady. The current lack of quality of vision is merely an inconvenience. No longer does it weigh down my day-to-day functioning.

The response to visual stimuli gradually improved. I contribute that to the passing of time and brain training. Time cannot be influenced, but brain exercises speed up cognitive performance and complement the recovery of vision. I do not participate in traffic. It goes too fast for me. My hesitation would be a danger to others.

A year after the stroke, I ordered new glasses for reading and distance. The prescription had changed drastically. A recent eye exam revealed further changes. The difference in measurement was too big to attribute solely to getting older. Apparently, the eyes continue adjusting.

Coordination

I always kept a "To-Do List." It gave me the feeling of being in control. For years, inventorying action points had reduced stress at work and helped me to get the most out of my spare time in my private life. I had never regarded loading my memory with trivial items as making good use of the brain; that is a task for the daily planner or PDA. Besides, I love the feel of having been productive when ticking off items. The review of the long list in memory would have been a waste too; you never know what you've forgotten.

In the hospital, it would come in handy to have my reminders at hand to pass on. My brain had enough to deal with, and there would be fewer loose ends in our communication. People had trouble understanding my speech; the voice was an unclear whisper. Working with notes would make life easier for everybody. At least, that is what I thought. I was fooling myself by trying to take command. For what-to-bring or who-to-call, I depended entirely on Dorthe; she was the one in charge. It merely polished up my self-esteem.

I picked up a pen and a piece of paper. Something had come to mind. The pen strokes were undecipherable; astonished, I inspected the pen and waved my hand at the pulse to check it was still there. I tried again and again. Painstakingly slowly, a single character appeared on paper; seconds later, another. This was not going to work.

I could read, with difficulty, but that is beside the point; I knew what the characters looked like and could rattle off the alphabet. They just would not appear on paper the way I envisioned them. To my amazement, I could no longer write.

Foremost, it was a matter of hand-eye coordination. My movements lacked precision, smoothness, and tempo. Yet, there was more to the problem than that: my poor eyesight complicated things. With one eye closed, the head slightly tilted, and the tongue between my lips, I jotted down a few words and gave up. The effect was comparable to the printer being out of order; the computer still worked but the output device failed. To make things worse, the webcam had problems too. It was frustrating, but it did not matter right now. When she arrived, Dorthe would patiently go through the effort of listening to what I meant to say. By now, she was used to my soft rasping voice, but the need to master my writing skills had gone up the ladder of priorities. New shortcomings reveal themselves over time. That is what makes rehabilitation an adventure. The challenge is fixing them when encountered. It would take the time it takes; there was no need to get bored.

That same day, I asked Dorthe to bring me a notebook. In my best possible handwriting, I constructed numbers and spelled out the alphabet and a choice words: 'Alpha,' 'Bravo,' 'Charlie.' Slowly my calligraphy came on paper. One exercise series, one page, each dated. The hour quickly passed. Slowly, the unwanted slanting of the words dipping below or jumping above the lines lessened. Thinking up words became a mental test. Different themes appeared on different pages: city names, countries, animals, or whatsoever. Psychologists would have found a wealth of material for associative analyses on the pages filled day-by-day.

I was back in my days at primary school. Suddenly I was that little boy again, back in class with the teacher in front of the chalk and blackboard; we meticulously copied her awe-inspiring handwriting. Long forgotten memories returned: the triple-lined sheets of paper, ink spots when the crown pen stuck to the cheap fibers, and the sweet taste of a blue tongue from wetting the tip of the pen as if it were a slate-pencil. The reward for hard work was to go around with a big flask of royal blue ink to refill the inkpots with their Bakelite sliding covers. No wonder old memories returned. Reprogramming my handwriting called for the same concentration, precision, and repetition it took to learn how to write in the first place.

The mornings were excellent for my little exercise. In between the routine early morning visits at my bedside by the hospital staff and the start of the day's schedule, I asked the nurse to take me down to the community room in my wheelchair. A small bag with necessities was fixed to the armrest: a pen, the book, and my mobile phone. Comfortably placed at the table in my pajamas, with the stand for the infusion next to me, I would unpack and start my work: because a job it was. It got me out of bed and in a different ambience. Suddenly my world was getting bigger. Working among other patients, the first social elements were creeping back in my life.

Re-learning the precise movements required patience and concentration. When the notebook was full, which took me a month, I could write again. I had re-learned the skill. The time it takes is not important as long as you can recognize progress. Records can be set on an interval basis: a day, a week, or a month. It was motivating to page back and forth and see the improvements; often, I took two steps forward and one step back. Not every page was necessarily better looking than the previous. From beginning to end, there was a difference of night and day. My first grade teacher would have been proud of me.

Nobody pays tribute to his talent anymore when hastily scribbling notes, but we should. We do many marvelous things without blinking an eye. When forced into rehabilitation, you quickly start to realize the complex interaction between mind and body; the efforts behind our abilities are amazing.

Karine took me shopping at the local supermarket in the tiny mall. Alone or accompanied by a therapist, many patients bought their little extras there. To the shop was only a short walk. Nonetheless, it was nice to get away from the hospital, and it was good exercise.

Karine's job as occupational therapist was to create self-sufficiency for functioning in everyday life. Motor coordination is essential for that. From our morning routine to setting the alarm for the night, we perform deceptively intricate tasks. Even the most trivial actions are the result of a complex interaction between body, brain, and senses. Without basic hand-eye coordination, most of us would be unable to perform even the simplest things; preparing a sandwich or flipping pages of a book would be difficult. Most instruments are complicated to play, and you need many lessons—even with a talent for it. There is room for optimism; our coordination gets better with exercise. Just as I relearned how to write, we can all learn to master and re-master.

Occupational therapists work at the cross-road of our mental, physical, and psychological abilities. Add to that the social element—living situation and special interests—and the occupational therapist can begin to contemplate what it takes the patient to live his life to its fullest. Finding solutions starts with understanding the problems. Optimizing the patient's potential is a rewarding profession. Likewise, so is the patient's job to rehabilitate.

The OT department was nicely equipped with a workshop, handy craft section, testing material, game room, and several small kitchens. Karine was creative in finding ways to achieve her goals, and used the facilities well. She had readily understood that I was more interested in doing something meaningful as opposed to following the traditional approach of sticking pins in a wooden tablet. The latter had actually revealed that my pincer-grip and hand-eye coordination were not up to standard. As we returned from our shopping trip with pounds of Norwegian prawns, she gave me a new assignment: "Why don't you start peeling. I'll see you shortly." Happily seated at one of the kitchen tables, I turned on the radio and started. Hours later, she apologetically rushed in, only to burst out in laughter at seeing a huge pile of prawns. I had met my quota for the day.

As soon as the news got out that I was an asset and not a liability, useful work came my way: a bicycle of one of the children of the nurses needed an overhaul, there were skis to wax, and the workshop manager had a backlog of maintenance work. All of the jobs had their challenges, and I enjoyed the feel of mastering more and more, little by little. A bit of renovation here, a bit of tinkering there: it taught me that everything you do is an exercise in its own right. You learn from your actions and reactions: how to maintain balance when applying force, plan a work sequence, or test your level of comprehension on a new recipe or technical instruction. Training for everyday life is found in everyday life.

The travel back and forth to the rehabilitation hospital was not easy for Dorthe. Due to the location of Sunnaas on a peninsula, it was a long detour in the busy commuter traffic. On the other hand, the travel by bus and ferry took less than an hour; what's more, I loved the passage across the icy waters of the fjord in the low winter sun. As the crow flies, it was a short distance home. The decision was easy. I would use public transportation for the weekend travel, and Dorthe would drive to the hospital once or twice during the week. The area and means of transportation were new to me. It was more than anybody could have ever asked for when Karine seized the therapeutic opportunity and accompanied me on the travel. She helped my little trolley through the snow, got me on board the bus, and took a seat with her colleagues. I was on my own, undertaking something that was major to me. Mentally, it had taken a lot of planning: what and how to pack, having money at hand in the right pocket, remembering the timetable, the walk to the bus, boarding with the crowd, buying the ticket, recalling where to get off, and having enough time to do so. It seems easy, but it had occupied my mind for the whole day. Every step had been premeditated. From a distance, Karine kept an eye on me. I felt independent and comfortably safe under her hidden supervision. She would bail me out—but only if necessary.

Besides training, the focus of OT is on establishing a positive mind-set, a can-do attitude, and methods to improve one's functioning to fit specific interests. Rebuilding confidence in the functioning of the patient is something that will be a continuous process. It goes beyond formal rehabilitation. It is important to understand how to keep up progress and what inspires. When at ease with designing your personal exercises, try to develop new functions or broaden existing ones. It is good to create, but sometimes temper, your expectations.

Compliments are important motivators. For the patient it is good to get positive feedback on his accomplishments. After all, he labored hard, and it is stimulating to get recognition. The pride of mastering new functions is a strong incentive to keep up the good work.

In the context of rehabilitation, my definition of coordination provides an indication of mastering fine and crude movements related to motor functions as a percentage of pre-stroke competence.

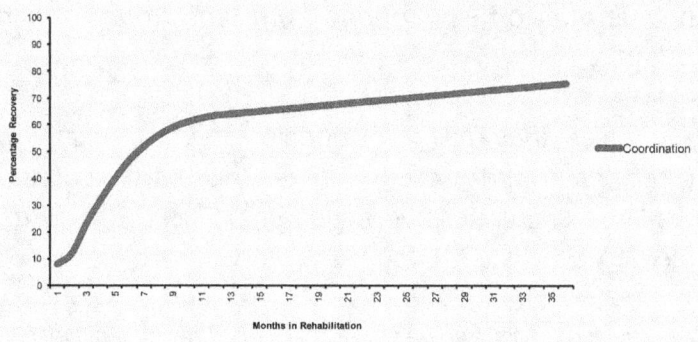

Figure 6. Coordination

Coordination of movements was seriously troubled by other factors during the early phase of medical recovery. Restrictions on vision, muscle strength, energy, and concentration prohibited any significant attempts.

Coordination is dependent on the integration of many different physical, sensory, and neurological functions. It was not until I was out of the medical doldrums that I understood the actual boundaries. The first practical sign of having lost the ability to control my fine movements was when I tried to make some notes. The pen would not flow over the paper as I wanted it to. With training, I have solved that problem. Once in the upswing of recovery, old routines eventually became smoother, more precise, and less time consuming; simply put, less clumsy.

During my time at the rehabilitation hospitals, the coordinative abilities improved steeply. Fewer early limitations were holding me back. After approximately one year, two-thirds of my ability returned. That is good enough to get by in normal life as long as you have the chance to do things at your own pace and people offer a helping hand from time to time when asked.

I feel that being incapable of multitasking in combination with my sensitivity to stress and my quickly depleted energy reserve negatively influenced a faster recovery.

Over the last two years of recovery, I regained most of my ability to coordinate my motor-dependent functions. The recovery of my coordination is roughly in line with the average of the other medical, mental, and physical key areas.

Nowadays, what influences my ability most is not the coordination of movements itself— doing things properly—but of other functions that are closely related. Actions fail to go smoothly when I am too tired, pushed for time or results, or asked to flip on a coin. Being aware of what impacts coordination negatively helps you to arm yourself against the cause.

Physical Strength

The plaster came off. In six weeks, the muscle mass had visibly shrunk: a thin white leg next to the one that was tanned and strong. There was no need to worry; the X-ray was good, and my strength would return quickly. Soon, I would walk again with the same old energetic pace.

That was years ago. My loss of physical strength after the stroke was different. Instantaneously, an overall weakness had set in. It went beyond sheer muscle power. To get up from the sofa, I needed both arms to push me up or stretch out for help. As if filtered out, the muscles lacked any neural sense of urgency to work for it. My movements were slow and weak, and they needed contemplation. Motion and force lacked momentum; the impetus was gone.

Once discharged from hospital, I did not live by the routine of an institution anymore. My day used to revolve around an agenda set by therapists. There was a rigid moment for everything from getting up to dinnertime, with exercises and power naps sandwiched in. Following the schedule guaranteed a day full of activity. At home, life was very different. Suddenly, I had to set my own agenda. Then, at a certain point, I had to function without special support.

The service of the health system is confined. Fair enough, I had spent about nine months in hospitals, and the resources are limited. Dismissed to make room for the next patient, my overall recovery was halfway. I was no longer dependent on others but far from capable of performing my daily routines with confidence. My strong points in recovery had been my vision and swallowing. The weak points were handling stress, multitasking, and using my voice. They would require daily practice over time, and for the voice, a simple operation. In the mid-range, my physical strength, energy, balance, and coordination needed a lot of additional work.

Dorthe and I would have to manage the return to society ourselves. We had our work orders: make physical exercising a priority; the body will not start to perform better without it. Training would require perseverance and ultimate precision. It would be hard work but an easy commitment. There was no choice; I owed family, friends, and myself. The gym was an obvious place to start reconditioning mind and body.

Find a gym where you feel comfortable. The nicest is to find a place that is within reach by foot or bicycle. A nearby location reduces the threshold of a visit and the short trip outdoors will add to the exercise. Fitness centers aimed at all ages are a better match than those that provide a second home to bodybuilders. Some of the superior facilities have a swimming pool or spa with a lounge or fruit bar. These bells and whistles can offer you some reward after the training. The prospect of relaxing in the whirlpool, resting under the solarium, or treating yourself to a freshly squeezed orange juice may be the incentive that makes you look forward to your visits. When in Spain, Dorthe and I found our post-training relaxation spot in a nearby cafe. Soon we became regulars at Terraza Aguadulce where we treated ourselves to the luxury of a light breakfast, a morning newspaper, and the time to let the training efforts sink in.

Technical facilities of the gym are of course what counts and not the bonus afterwards. A good fitness center offers support by personal trainers. Using their expertise once-or-twice a week is an excellent way to get started. After an initial talk to discuss health, condition, and objectives, they will prepare a personal training and nutrition plan. Furthermore, the trainers will explain which equipment is appropriate and how to use it, and they will coach you during the exercises. Attention to the psyche is vital. There are feelings of insecurity to overcome before self-confidence returns. A good PT will coach rather than instruct and focus on the combination of mental and physical aspects to achieve results. After a few months, you should be able to continue on your own accord or reduce the frequency of active support by your PT. It depends on your goals, which will most likely change in line with your progress and personal economy.

Most fitness centers offer a wide range of group lessons such as spinning, aqua gym, and aerobics. The gym may offer group lessons in relaxation as well. The classes are typically included in the membership and worth a try. There is always something to gain. Beside the physical part, you may benefit from a fixed time for working out, which adds to the training discipline, or appreciate the social value. The lessons may be targeted at improving the overall physical condition, balance, coordination, or strength. It is important to follow at your own pace. Do not to dismiss the opportunity of attending group lessons too quickly. There is a learning curve for everything. Explain to the instructor what your challenges are, and you will most certainly get that little bit of extra attention.

Training is effective at any level but only as long as you use the right technique and give it your best. There are no shortcuts. Not all exercises should be performed at your physical limits. In general, the combination of load and repetitions matters. Working with lesser weights or a lower resistance can be equally effective if the frequency or duration of the exercise is increased. One of my favorite classes was spinning. Nobody but me decided how much friction to put on the flywheel. Everything is relative; as long as you sweat for it, you will be doing as good as the "pros".

Relaxation training focuses on the inner relations between mind and body. Deepening the awareness of your functions with slow and precise movements supports the fine-tuning of balance, coordination, and breathing and relieves muscle tension. Given the usual effects of a stroke, it makes sense to include relaxation training in the weekly schedule. Stretching, yoga, and pilates are excellent ways to counterbalance the body stress of the tougher physical exercises.

There is always the temptation to skip training. Excuses to let it pass for the day are easy to stumble on. Once you are out of the rhythm, it is hard to pick it up again. The next time around, the exercises will be tougher. Those hardships will reduce your enthusiasm, and motivation will suffer. Make training a priority in life. Mind and body need it more than ever. When I dropped out for a while, I quickly noticed a setback in my recovery. Therefore, make your workout a pleasant experience, pick a comfortable environment, and set up weekly plans. Decide on the best time of the day, and plan your training sessions accordingly. A fixed appointment with a PT will help to establish the training discipline.

An excellent way of not being tempted to bail out is to find a training partner who is willing and able to share your commitment. With a bit of mutual loyalty, you can pull each other through on days when one happens to lack the drive. Remember, even when you were not quite up to it, it was a great feeling to have completed your training program. Afterward, the accomplishment is something nobody can take away. Then you can treat yourself to that well-deserved bonus.

The physical effects are quickly noticeable when working out every other day for an hour or two. A higher frequency will not do you much good unless there is adequate variation in the training routine. Focus each session on different objectives: cardio or aerobic, upper-body or legs, balance or strength. There was a period when I saw an exercise in everything. It was a nasty side effect of too much concentration for too long. Rehabilitation had become more than a full-time job. Keeping up the motivation was a challenge. I needed to give the brain time to recuperate.

When occupied with fun and play, it is easier to bring the autopilot back to life. Indoor exercises tend to get boring. Fortunately, there is a world outdoors waiting to be explored. Riding my bicycle, playing a ball game, or splashing in the pool with kids was what I needed. A child's perception of life is uncomplicated; seek their participation. Their playfulness will rub off on you.

The common view is that people are considered healthy as long as they are not ill. However, confronted with an unhealthy situation and after a bit of thought, it is easy to realize that the true meaning of 'health' is the fine balance between physical abilities and mental well-being. Working out not only improves the condition, but increases one's mental strength. Regular exercise reduces the vulnerability to negative stress. Overtraining can cause injury and deplete the energy reserve. Do not let blunt stubbornness obscure the consequences. To continue exercising when overly tired will not improve the results. On the contrary, it will take the body much longer to recuperate and undermine your training ability and therefore, the motivation.

The concentration to perform creates a constant mental pressure. That load consumes lots of energy. Make sure that you rest well before doing your fitness routine. Learning how to regulate the use of energy so that you get pleasure from working strength, coordination, and balance is something that takes time. Just like the body, the mind needs time to restore its form. Training longer and harder is not necessarily better as the total well-being may suffer and the motivation will be short lived. Short pauses between exercises and longer intervals between training sessions improve the results.

After a while, I learned to identify my physical flaws more accurately. Inventive thinking with a twist of common sense helped in the design of exercises to target those weak points; after that, I set clear objectives and worked toward achieving them pragmatically. To reduce my sway when walking, I worked the cross machine with my eyes closed. The slightest variation in muscle tension immediately signaled any need for correction to the brain. It raised a few eyebrows, but people could tell that I was seriously working on something that mattered to me. Soon, respect for my persistence replaced their questioning looks. Within a month, my balance had drastically improved. The large rooms, normally used for group training, offered privacy and were of use to practice skipping rope or trying balancing acts. Large mirrors on the wall provided positive feedback.

In the beginning, it was much easier to master forgotten abilities. Starting to work on the evident shortcomings first and taking on the fine points later was the obvious thing to do. However, it is typically the last twenty percent that takes as long as the first eighty. Breaking records motivates, but when it begins to take longer to achieve your goals, changing to measuring partial progress is more appealing. For example, when skipping, with a final goal of thirty jumps in thirty days, you could take the best daily score out of three tries. Working your way up the ladder makes it competitive and is definitely more fun. Once you meet your goal, move on to the next challenge.

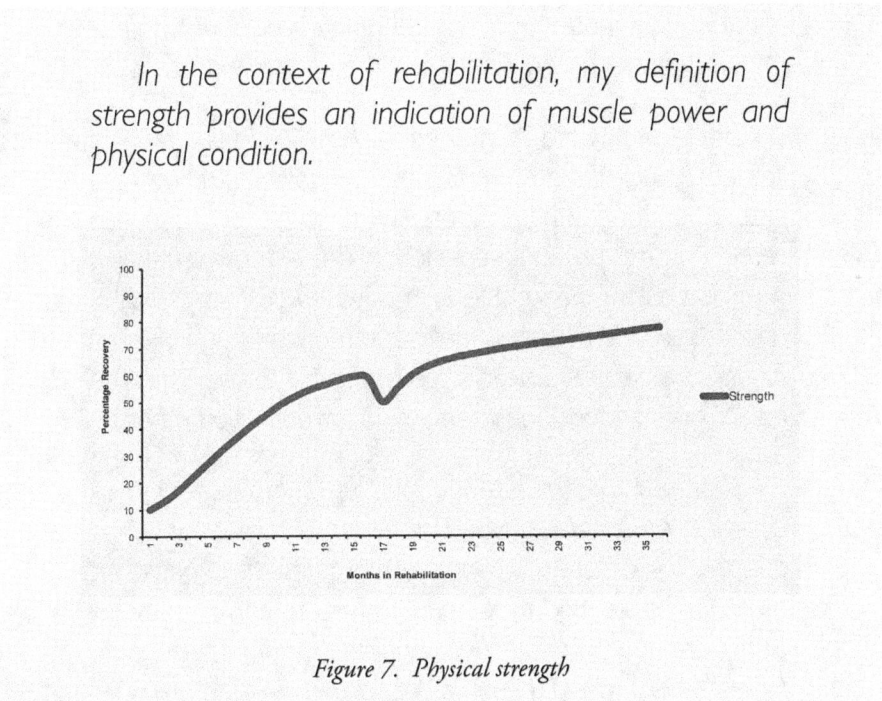

In the context of rehabilitation, my definition of strength provides an indication of muscle power and physical condition.

Figure 7. Physical strength

My strength was marginal after the stroke. Medically restrained by infusions and without any energy to spare, I could not picture myself in the gym. Learning how to walk, talk, and eat was on top of my agenda. Then there was my mobility and double vision to deal with. No, my mind was not on physical training. I would deal with that when I was ready for it. I had enough on my mind to bother its limited capacity with yet another task.

It was not until the swallowing disorder was mended and my energy level increased that my physical weakness surfaced. As I started my walking exercises, the first physical training came into my life. I moved stealthily through the hospital corridors. Once I had overcome my fear for the steep descent, I kept practicing going up and down the stairs. Although never far from a handrail, I regained my mobility. During rehabilitation, about half of my strength returned. After that, the recovery flattened.

Being motivated is one thing; how to keep it up is something else. I tried to take a break halfway through the second year, and within a month, I was experiencing a serious setback in my physical condition and mental well-being. It was particularly noticeable in my walking, stress handling, and coordination. I should not have reduced my workouts. During my stay in Spain, I focused on a combination of indoor and outdoor training. It gave my motivation a boost.

Currently, I would rate my level of physical strength as acceptable. However, this is on the condition that I have say over the kind of activity and time of execution, the expectation of performance, and that I am allowed to complete tasks at my own tempo. This equally applies to shopping, a bicycle tour, or work around the house or garden.

Balance

Not long after the turn of the millennium, the company Segway unveiled the Personal Transporter. Its first production model, a self-balancing scooter, entered the market a year later. The piece of equipment could have come straight out of a science fiction movie: futuristic, robotic, silent, green, and magical. The driver stands on a small platform between two parallel wheels and holds onto a handlebar. The movement of the vehicle reacts to body sway: forward, stop, left, and right. It is simple and intuitive. Traffic lawmakers did not have a clue how to classify the device. By now, balancing scooters are walkway-legal in most countries. Perhaps seen as a gadget at first, with the official blessings in place, the Personal Transporter may well gain widespread acceptance amongst able-bodied and disabled people alike.

The balance technology of the device is based on angular rate sensors and accelerometers that sense changes in the terrain and the driver's body position in a fraction of a second. Although limited when compared to balancing the human body, there is an analogy with our biomechanics. We are created to do more than just move and turn—and often under very demanding circumstances. Maintaining our balance is constantly challenged: from when we get dressed to turning in. With every step we take, our sensors adjust our balance mechanism; in the dark or in bright daylight, on a slope or on one foot, we manage to stay upright. When we are pushed, we push back. If we fall, we get up.

In biomechanics, balance is the ability to maintain the center of mass of the body within the base of support with minimal sway. To do so, the biological system provides the brain with a continuous stream of signals from the inner ear, muscle movement, and other senses. Like the Segway gyros, the labyrinth in the inner ear monitors both direction and acceleration of motion. The eyes monitor how we are positioned and where we are heading. The touch of our feet provides the central nervous system with information about the terrain and the distribution of our gravity load. Meanwhile, the muscle and joint sensory receptors report body movements. Add intentions, and the brain has the daunting task to process all those bits of information simultaneously and come up with a coordinated response. Our biomechanics are superior to anything manmade but equally vulnerable to faults. If any of the sensors fail, or if the brain is not up to speed, it results in imbalance.

My balance was a problem from day one. The laws of gravity were ignored as the ambulance silently made its way through town; strapped to the stretcher, I could not tell up from down. Months later, I still had that same experience as soon as my eyes lost track of the horizon or when I lay down too abruptly. For comfort and safety, I made sure that the side racks of the hospital bed where properly locked in the upright position. My seemingly weightless rolls became part of life and slowly lost some of their initial scare.

My sensors were no longer reliable. Some needed active training; others, passive healing over time. Double vision hindered a proper survey of my surroundings. The feeling of touch and pressure was flawed, which made it difficult to determine the distribution of body weight. My muscle coordination was slow; the brain would go through a dress rehearsal prior to every action. The sensor in the inner ear needed calibration. With every abrupt move, I felt lost in space. Most importantly, the brain's little super computer could not make sense out of the garbled sets of data it was receiving, let alone issue the right instructions to counter any physical disturbances. Processing the data in a matter of milliseconds would require a lot of re-engineering. I was in for a long haul. It was going to be a big project, but I was determined to succeed.

I would not trust a two-legged table, and a four-legged table, although usually safe, is never in perfect balance. Only a three-legged table will never wiggle due to a solvable equation of the equilibrium. Laws of physics or mechanical calculations are not the topic here, but I want to share a practical observation. If you have problems with balancing on both legs, touching a third point with a fingertip, with not more than a few grams of force, can solve the whole balance equation in a snapshot. That is why a walking cane can make such a difference, and there is no need to lean heavily on it either. The opportunity was lost on me; my wife had told me unambiguously that using a walking stick was out of the question. No walking aids meant going back to my exercises.

Sometimes training goes beyond the regular boundaries. I exercised on indoor climbing walls during my rehabilitation several times. One thing is certain: they are diverse and definitely fun. To my surprise, climbing a vertical wall was far from the scary experience I had expected. With good instructions and a bit of daredevilry, you can make it to the top. I had not expected such strong positive feelings afterward. Balance was not an issue. Beginners typically have two feet and one hand, or two hands and one foot, on the protrusions. The three-point contact with the wall must have eliminated the difficulties with my balance. The constant tension on the safety line kept me secure and provided an opportunity to take a rest and plan the next move. I realized that my strength left a lot to be desired, but otherwise, the exercise was a big hit. The sensation of mastering something as exotic as wall climbing was the high point of the day.

The good old autopilot had made me forget the simplest things about balance and the way I moved. Practicalities were lost in memory: What is the easiest way to get up from the floor? When the left leg moves forward, is it the right or left arm that swings along? Did I dress standing up or sitting down? How long could I stand on one leg…and with my eyes closed? The complexity of our actions is striking.

Just as a baby learns to crawl and stand, fall and get up, you can improve your balance by training. The big difference is that infants learn to walk out of a playful curiosity. Their focus is not on the movement itself but on the target: a toy or an unattended pot of chocolate sauce on the kitchen counter. Adults who relearn walking do not have the patience and analyze every step of the way.

The second time around, we learn the basics; the primary focus of the physiotherapists is on how we walk, not why. It is serious training; the emphasis is no longer on the playful aspect or the reward at our destination but on the technique. With one exception though. At the rehabilitation hospital, we ended our morning gymnastics with some simple fun. The aim of the game was to keep a beach ball airborne as long as possible by playing one-to-the-other while counting the strikes aloud: "...six, seven, eight...." On the soft mat, I moved quickly to ready myself for a nice return: "...nine,ten,eleven...." All of a sudden, I lunged toward the ball and played the most beautiful volley: "... twelve, thirteen...." The game element had triggered a subconscious reflex; for a split second, the excitement had surpassed the tempo of my analytical mind. The experience of losing myself in the thrill of the moment taught me a few things: training has to be diverse and fun, and children make good therapists.

Many deficiencies after a stroke are hard to quantify and the recovery process can be slow. Having an absolute reference to measure recovery is valuable. The occupational therapist confirmed what I had suspected, but now she was able to put a number on it. The test, which revolved around touching the skin with thin hairs of different stiffness, while having to guess the spot she probed, was objective. The sensitivity of half my body was coarse. The limited feel in the soles of my feet added to my balance problems. I experienced an exclusive phenomenon: how it is to walk on clouds...wobbly.

Strangely enough, the skin of the affected parts of the body registered temperature with a different scale. My build-in thermometer worked; I could differentiate between hot and cold. What I touched with the inferior side felt different; cold felt colder, and warm felt cooler. The scale must have been off by ten degrees centigrade. The erroneous effect seems to have lessened over time, and I have learned to live with the inconvenience. Actually, some make-believe resistance to heat does have benefits in the kitchen.

The swimming pool at the rehabilitation hospital was a tempting test bed for my balance. What would be the reaction of mind and body to sensing the water temperature with disparity? Would a shivering half of me want to flee quickly from the heated pool? My feel for balance had improved, but I could expect a total loss of orientation. Moving almost weightless in three dimensions would most certainly be a major challenge. It took some time to explain to the staff why I wanted to submit myself to the test. Hesitant at first, their curiosity won. Together with the therapist and with the guard on stand-by beside the pool, I was allowed to look for answers. Sometimes the direct approach is the best way to create an understanding. Carefully, I stepped into the unknown. Rehabilitation is an adventure, and everything you learn helps you to respond better to the challenges ahead. I am an optimist at heart but also a realist; I was mentally prepared for a fresh list of exercises before making a second attempt.

To my disbelief, body and mind responded as normal. My body experienced the water temperature as one-and-the-same. Carried by the water, I could swim easier than I could walk. My muscle coordination was smooth, and the movement was light. I managed to swim underwater and turn without losing my orientation. No wet roller coaster ride as I managed turns and a swim on my back. Swimming gave moving around a new dimension. Enclosed by water, the brain seemed capable of filtering the ambiguous sensory input to interpret the body's whereabouts correctly. After this positive experience, I am convinced about the usefulness of water gymnastics in rehabilitation.

As I was getting out of my swimsuit, I set myself a new goal: getting dressed standing up. Trying to keep my balance on one foot would be entertaining. I had tested the theory for weeks in the evenings when roaming the hospital. Standing still under the clock in the lobby, I found my balance, waited for the second-hand to reach twelve, and slowly lifted one leg, concentrated, and adjusted my sway. Eventually, I managed to keep it up for almost a full minute. To counteract the difficulty with my vision, I had placed a small sticker on the pillar as a focal point. To succeed, I concentrated so hard on that stable point that the wall almost gave way. A quick glimpse at the clock in between would abruptly break off the exercise.

The physiotherapist had just explained that I was not standing straight but slanted to the right. Oddly enough, I was convinced otherwise but did not dare to challenge her observation. It took me an hour in front of the big mirror in the gym to create the awareness. The method gave me an idea of how to go about the fix. I closed my eyes; now without the sensory input of my vision, my brain was working hard trying to interpret the weight that I placed on each foot, the muscle tension, and slight swing of the body. Slowly, I opened my eyes. The door frame behind me gave me a useful reference. Yes, of course, she was correct; my posture was off by a few degrees. Just straightening my shoulders would not remedy the problem.

The next few days, I spent many hours in front of the mirror: close your eyes, lean forward, backward, sideways, and straighten until vertical; open your eyes, and check the result. It must have been a strange view for the other patients to see me doing seemingly nothing in utmost concentration. Whatever people might have thought, I knew that I could learn to correct my balance by presenting an image to the brain that proved the error in the calculation. It was like debugging line after line of computer code. The process required endless repetition, but I made steady progress. The finishing touches to reinstating my sense of balance needed many small steps, each consuming lots of time and energy. This was just one of them. A week later this particular job was done.

Walking

In Norwegian, the walking-aid is called a *prekestol*; the direct translation would be 'cancel.' Factually, it is a walking frame: a tall tubular U-shaped construction open at the back, with four small wheels at the bottom corners. The top side is covered with a leather patch to lean on with when standing inside. The young physiotherapist helped me out of bed and into my 'cancel.' She held onto the frame to stop it from running off—ready to grab me—and led me slowly forward. I coped and slippered over the floor while heavily leaning on the armrests. Together, we conquered the length of the corridor, taking a rest every few meters. I smiled broadly from ear to ear. I had to show this to the boys and call my wife to tell her about my first steps.

It was incredibly motivating. The sensation had awakened the slumbering willpower to actively influence my healing and take control. Determined to beat record-upon-record, I worked the corridors up and down, day and night if I could. This was only the beginning. The outlook for the future suddenly seemed so much brighter. Not just for that first walk, but also because I had found something tangible to fight.

I had seen babies moving around in colorful plastic walking chairs. Eventually they learned to walk, so why not me? There was no loss of control over my limbs. It reduced relearning to training. Irrespective of the barriers ahead, I would walk again: been there, done that. The second time around, my learning curve should be steeper. I looked forward to the daily sessions. To my impatience, I had the weekends off but continued practicing alone or with my visitors. The pressure on my legs gradually increased; I now stood and lifted my feet. Triumphant, I measured my successes by distance: to the end of the corridor, the lounge, or all the way to the main hall.

I entered the period of beating one personal record after the other. Under the appreciative eye of the staff, I endlessly repeated what I had learned. Their compliments fueled my motivation. In the evening hours, I demonstrated for Dorthe what I had managed. The two of us became regulars in the hospital corridors when working the exercises in a double shift. My spirits were in an upswing. These were exciting times. The adventure of rehabilitation had eventually started.

The exercises for walking without support began in the quiet corridors of Diakonhjemmet hospital. With the therapist on one side and in reach of a long bar mounted to the wall on the other, I made my first steps under my own steam. We counted strides until I would grab one or the other. The pause eased the positive tension. Happily, we would prepare for yet another lap, and another. My first steps were rigid—like the human-like C-3PO, the buddy of little R2-D2 in the movie *Star Wars*—with arms and legs jolting and feet just a little too wide apart. Robotic or not, I was marching: left–right, left–right, chest forward, joints locked, arms too noticeably in sync.

Taking the stairs was an entirely different challenge. Looking down the flight of steps, even when holding on to the handrail, was frightening; was I really up to this? Uneasy, I descended and carefully listened to the comments on technique and posture. It took comparatively long to get it right. Switching my weight from foot to foot or skipping the intermediate step and alternate the stride for each tread was nerve-racking. Eventually, I mastered the third dimension.

The atmosphere was good. Others had witnessed the cheerful turnaround. People felt involved; it was stimulating. When your world is too small for too long, it is easy to succumb to lethargy and become indifferent and insensitive toward people. On the opposite side, wider surroundings inspire communication, involvement, and enthusiasm. Mobility meant that I was no longer dependent on others to explore the social opportunities available.

Here is a survey for you: take a seat on a terrace on a sunny afternoon, order a beer, and observe the way people walk. Soon, you will realize how many people wiggle and wobble, drag their feet, strike the ground with their toes pointed outward, and never complete a roll from heel to toe.

It is astonishing how few people actually go by the book. Applying the proper technique is one of the things I am very conscious about. Not because of the looks, but walking properly makes optimal use of kinetic, potential, and elastic energy in the pendulum swing. In short, it makes going by foot lighter, durable, and pleasurable. The good news is that even with a bad technique, it is not that difficult to blend in with the crowd.

An athlete racewalking at the Olympics must always have one foot on the ground. The walker is disqualified for running if both feet are seen in the air. Different bio-mechanics distinguish walking from running. Anyhow, I would be happy enough with a nice stroll around the block. During a normal walk, the leg swings forward from the hip; the foot touches the ground with the heel and rolls through to the toe in a smooth motion. The opposite arm swings along. The energy of the bounce is temporarily stored in the muscles—like in a squeezed rubber ball—to be released again when the leg stretches to pass under the body. The center of mass is raised and drops as the legs are spread. It is easy to see what is happening when you simulate a walk with two fingers in slow motion over the tabletop and look at your knuckles.

Spring in Oslo was only in attendance on the calendar. Roads were icy between white walls left by the snowplows. Nevertheless, with a steel-pointed stick in hand and my eyes protected against the cold wind by sunglasses, I loved being outdoors with Dorthe. She would take me on short trips downtown for a double espresso at Bocato or check out the shopping malls at Aker Brygge.

Crossing the street was demanding. First, regaining my balance when making the mandatory stop at the curb; next, judging the traffic: turn the body, look left, see that a car is approaching, determine its speed, estimate how long will it take to get here, look right, look left again, observe that the car is closer. My little built-in calculator tried to do the arithmetic to determine safe passage until deciding that a better-safe-than-sorry approach was in my best interest. After all, pulling a short sprint in case my assessment was wrong was not in the cards. I preferred the protection of a zebra crossing to the danger of an unreliable guess, and I was more than willing to make a little detour to get to a pedestrian-safe zone.

When I walk, I walk, and when I talk, I talk; the need to concentrate ruled out doing two things at the same time. Single-tasking was tricky enough. I lived in one dimension: no jaywalking or taking shortcuts. A delay in observation and thought forced all actions in sequence. What used to be the result of the subconscious now came in discrete steps, each contemplated and rigidly analyzed until decided upon. The inability to multitask had irritating effects throughout. I quickly developed a simple technique to hide the shortcoming from others and myself. When entering a large space or meeting a crowd, I would buy some time by making a strategic stop, study the setting, and say to my companion; "Nice place. Where would you like to go next?" while checking for obstacles and planning my next move. Alas, Dorthe saw straight through my delay tactic but gracefully granted me the time to get ready to proceed.

Not all progress is the result of a deliberate effort. When crossing the square at the sea front, I took notice of the time on the clock of the eastern tower at city hall without a pause and picked up an envelope from the doormat while entering the apartment. The reflexes were a bonus to my training. The fact that I had not premeditated the trivial acts was promising.

The walks through town and the nearby countryside became longer. I took pleasure in the walks but could not let go of making it an exercise; relentlessly, I placed one foot in front of the other. I needed a diversion of the mind: something light-hearted. When my little nephew was visiting us in

101

Spain, I made a playful beginning by running against him for some nonsense reason. The beauty with small children is that running is about having fun and not winning or losing. Not judged on victory but on being a good sport, it opens a wealth of opportunity to slip in some practice through the back door.

The rehabilitation agenda sets itself. I found yet another challenge when Dorthe asked me to pick some fresh lemons. The Mediterranean cuisine uses many fruits, and the branches of the citrus trees in the garden were a clear evidence of that; the ripe ones were just out of reach. However hard I tried, I could not jump; my feet kept glued to the ground. What looks like a simple move is actually quite complex. After taking the proper starting position, a single burst of coordinated muscle action throws the body upward, in the midst of the ploy to grasp a ripe lemon, and then lands and recoups its balance. The next day I bought a jump rope at El Corte Inglés. As I read the directions for use—no one would ever have guessed that such a waiver existed for a piece of rope—I learned that there are many ways of using it. Techniques ranged from basic to very advanced. Without any ambition to become a pro, I decided to settle for the beginner level, make the exercise part of my fitness routine, and leave it at that. Within a few days, I could handle a dozen jumps. It never became my favorite activity and after a few weeks, I locked away the rope.

By now, I am back in Oslo, and I buy my lemons at the convenient store around the corner. The murky winter has fallen; the roads are covered with snow and slippery. On a cold and windy Saturday evening, Dorthe and I dressed up to dine at one of the trendy restaurants at the waterfront. Cuddled up, we came around the corner leading to the marina where a gust of wind blew off my brand new Borsalino. I froze in my steps. Helplessly, I watched my wide-rimmed Italian hat roll toward the dark icy water like tumbleweed. On high heels, Dorthe pulled a sprint and caught it just before it would have disappeared. Turning back with hat in hand, she was met by applause from a smiling audience from inside the corner restaurant. This summer I will be out in Vigeland Park to give jogging some more serious tries; maybe I'll combine it with a picnic and a game of soccer with the little ones.

People hardly notice my walking deficiencies any more. On the down side, I do not receive the many flattering remarks to which I have become accustomed. Being too cautious remains a thing to work on. I tend to move more careful than necessary when negotiating obstacles on my path, which is reflected in a sudden hesitant style of walking.

When shopping or going on a trip, walking is easier with a small backpack. Carrying a load is better done on the back than dragging along one or more shopping bags or a trolley. The weights create a sideways sway, which complicates maintaining balance. A backpack, on the other hand, improves the vertical posture. Walking straight improved the quality of my stride, and I could keep my hands free. The possibility to swing my arms along with each step or to grasp a handrail improved my sense of security, but sometimes I just want to hold hands.

In the context of rehabilitation, my definition of balance provides an indication of the development of mobility.

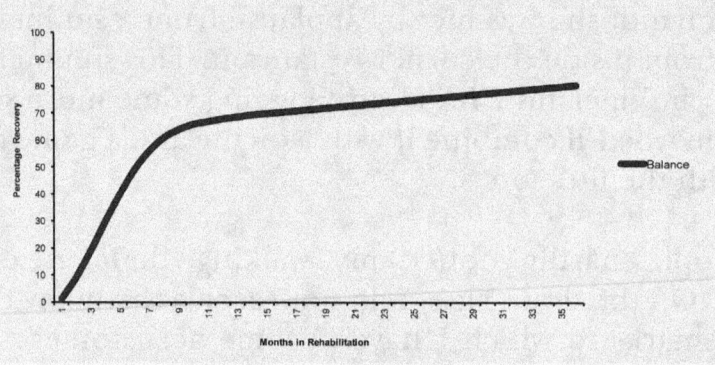

Figure 8. Balance and Walking

Two-thirds of my mobility restored within the first year. The level of advance in such a short lapse of time is spectacular by any measure. From being helped out of bed into a wheelchair to walking without aids has enormous practical impact on life. Without the constant need for assistance, it means getting up when you feel like it, going to the toilet alone, taking a shower, dressing yourself, and moving about freely. Not always having to ask is enough to return your feelings of independence. The freedom of mobility offers the opportunity to take your life back.

The recovery went up steeply immediately after the start of the balance and walking training and the progress did not flatten until the basics were in reasonable working order. From this phase onward, the advance became slow. By now, my balance suffers more from insecurity, stress or the lack of energy to sustain my stability over a longer period than anything else.

Fine-tuning the technique and the improvement of quality is demanding and time-consuming. The time between records slowed down from days to weeks and months. The duration to master a new task increased in line with the added complexity. It may call for a different approach to keep up your motivation. Consider the possibility of breaking down a complex task into a set of smaller events that are easy to measure. Above all, be prepared for a reduced tempo of recovery. Enjoy the lesser intensity with pride.

Often one learns about his or her shortcomings only when confronted. Some will never be discovered until challenged. Three years down the line, I still have my work spelled out: walk longer distances, hike in mountainous terrain, comfortably engage in a short run, and cope with a rolling deck aboard a small ship. Challenges are plentiful, and therefore, I do not rate my current recovery much higher than eighty percent.

Stress

The causes of stress and the stimuli for the different types of stress vary from person to person. I love sailing, and being at sea creates a positive stress. Somebody who is afraid of water and wiggly boats will hate it and experience the anxiety that comes with negative stress.

Stress is a mental state. It is created by the pressure to perform, self-induced or not, and the frustration of potential failure or inability. At least, that is the most common notion. Personally, I apply a further differential; there is positive and negative stress. Whereas negative stress is normally unhealthy, positive stress makes the adrenaline flow, and you perform better than you considered possible.

We cannot always avoid stress; in fact, sometimes we should not want to. Often, controlled stress gives a person the competitive edge in performance-related activities like sports, a hobby, or even work. Positive stress is your personal mental coach. It keeps you going with a smile at a level that creates respect.

The pressure to cook a gourmet dinner for friends in an unfamiliar kitchen will probably create negative stress. The pressure to be part of a team onboard a boat that is out there to win a regatta will most likely result in positive stress. Unless you are up to it, it is probably best to invite your friends out for dinner but not aboard a ship in a rough sea with a galley that you do not know very well.

Negative stress should be avoided and positive stress used to your advantage. The ability to deal with negative stress will have deteriorated after a brain stroke, while positive stress is something that can speed up recovery. The question to ask yourself with everything you undertake is: "Does it have the potential to increase frustration, or will it improve my motivation?"

Mental pressures that exceed your stress limits can cause considerable problems. Anxiety or a psychological blow will most likely disturb your functioning for quite some time. Worry, or emotional tension, is not the kind of thing you appreciate in normal life and not in the least when working on your recovery. Your emotions can rapidly turn into anger or an outcry of anxiety. There were many occasions where I must have stressed others as much as I stressed myself.

Distress causes biological responses of the body. Many signs are easy to recognize: an increased pulse, sweating, or muscle tension. Other symptoms are out of sight: increased blood pressure or a change in metabolism. A common effect of negative stress is the danger of an unstoppable slide down the spiral of mental self-control. Simply put, you lose it. One clumsy mistake leads easily to the next. It is Murphy's Law at work: "Anything that can go wrong will go wrong." An accident never comes alone.

Imagine yourself driving a car, and suddenly, things start to go wrong. The car behind you honks the horn and pushes you to hurry up. You ask yourself if you have overlooked something and re-evaluate the traffic situation. By the time you move, the light switches to red again, but you are already halfway on the crossing. Meanwhile, the windshield wipers screech from right to left because the horn made you jump and inadvertently touch the controls. A long truck makes a wide turn and almost rips open the left side of the car. A boy suddenly appears on your right and yells something at you—perhaps he is selling a newspaper or offering to wash your windshield, or maybe he is an upset pedestrian that you overlooked. Guaranteed, scoring three-out-of-three will make you want to quit or seriously lose your temper. Too bad but there is nowhere to go. Maybe there is a passenger to take it out on: good for you, bad for him. Admit it: you should not have been in this situation in the first place. A sequence of simple things may easily catch you off guard, and you realize that you are not stable enough to deal with the stress of the unexpected. Under those circumstances, take a time-out; take a deep breath, go back to the basics, and try again. Unless you master the technique, it is not easy to snap out of a stressful situation without the help of somebody who takes control on your behalf.

A good way to reduce negative stress is to exercise forward planning. Another is simply to do one thing at the time and stop overloading yourself by learning to say, "No." Be cautious though; there is a danger in becoming too questioning in everything you do. You lose the flexibility to flip on a coin.

If you commit to more than you are comfortable with, you run the risk of disappointing yourself as well as others. When you say, "Yes" to everything, it will increase the expectations of the people around you, and the threshold of your capability will quickly exceed your capacity. Worry and mental conflicts resulting in a constant switching between priorities are the result. When you recognize that your mind or coordination is struggling, try to reduce the workload. The best way to eliminate this type of stress is at the root. Simply putting a stop to it may raise some eyebrows initially, because it is not how people knew you, but they will quickly get used to it. I have taken a very drastic approach to cut back on the stress of multitasking: I do one thing at a time and finish it before taking on anything new. I found that by saying, "No, let me finish this first," it works out to the better for everybody.

Forward planning can be done at different levels. When you are out shopping, the situation is mentally less demanding when you go to a mall where you know your way around and bring a list of necessary groceries. This practical approach helps to avoid the frustration of regrets by the time you are back home. Loads of people rely on shopping lists rather than their memory. You may not have had to do so in the past, but by anticipating your actions, you will find that it frees up your mind for other things.

To perform a task smoothly, it will be easier when you think through the various steps you plan to take and prepare your path, tools, and material in advance. Freeing your brain from trivial tasks or interruptions in a work sequence can create a positive experience. Your shopping trips can become enjoyable time out—not a compulsory job, but rather a social event with time for a pleasant light lunch.

Verbal communication with external contacts may also create negative stress. It can be hard to predict the reaction of outsiders and follow sudden changes in verbal usage. That makes it tough to premeditate the course of a conversation.

The situation becomes tricky when you call customer service but rather than finding a willing ear, you are connected to someone who wriggles crisscross through every argument in the book and beyond in order to get the company out of your rightful claim. Honestly, I would not even dare to attempt that—at least not verbally. My speed of reasoning is not up to it, and the stress would be too much. For that reason, under complex circumstances, I prefer written communication to trying to solve things with a quick call. Generally speaking, a written argumentation is in a specific order rather than ad hoc. Things may take longer to resolve, but with my being a bit slow, time now works to my advantage. Another option is to brief a trusted relation and delegate the task. Both reduce negative stress.

Another stress factor that I experienced in the early recovery period was the feeling of being misunderstood and feeling unreasonable judgment of my behavior. Fair to say, I did not always understand my own behavior either. A lack of control over the intonation of speech makes it difficult to come across as intended; it is not always what you say, but how you say it, that can put people off. The voice is a large part of one's personality, and in my case, there was hardly any timbre left. Add to that a slow understanding, and you have the basic ingredients of a faltering communication. I could get very frustrated by not being able to express myself properly or swiftly find the correct response; in a quarrel, my emotions would overtake my verbal skills. It was quite embarrassing to stamp my foot like an infant when deprived of verbal power; at least there was nothing wrong with my body language. It is not a nice way to treat people you care for and who care for you. It takes time to recognize and learn to adjust your behavior. So, what do you do in the meantime, stop talking? No, become a better listener!

To avoid negative stress, it is essential that you understand what the causes are. It is true that avoiding a stressful event is not always possible. A head-on confrontation with the situation is sometimes the only way. Choose your approach carefully; the situation can be too difficult to handle or take too much of your energy. In such a case, it is better to call on a mediator to assist in solving the problem than trying to handle it in person. A stiff argument can cause negative stress over a longer period. Endless talks until late at night over an unfair, unreasonable, or indecent way that you have been treated will not do you much mental good. Your feelings may be correct, but is it worth the energy? Where is the benefit to your health and healing?

Anticipating the requirements associated with your actions will make life easier; although, improving on your flexibility may be something you have to work on afterward. It is important to know your limitations. That is not always easy. The borders of your capabilities will move constantly. You may not even be aware of your current limitations. You will not realize that you cannot run until you can walk.

One way to invoke positive stress is to focus on things that you were good at and enjoyed doing. If not feasible now, take small steps. With my balance, it is not wise for me to hang around on a ship's deck. Yet the sea pulls at me. For now, I have to restrict myself to the marina and help my friends to get their boats ready for a new season.

To experience a setback adds to your frustration and does not improve motivation. It may be that you used to enjoy playing the full eighteen holes on the golf course. Nowadays, your balance may prevent an even swing, and you will be better off with cart and caddie. Rather than an attempt to play the green, you might benefit more from spending your time training on the driving range with a well-briefed instructor and take it from there. Going back to basics, before you are forced, proves to be good practice in rehabilitation. By eliminating possible disappointments, a controlled start may turn potential negative stress to positive. Breaking down a large task to smaller ones gives you better control and allows you to find your limitations as you go along.

Once you are about to start or finish a task, it is nice if your environment cooperates. It could be that you have finished writing a letter on your computer; wouldn't it be nice if your network works, the printer is set up, there is paper in the drawer, and your ink cartridges are full? If not, it will most likely cause irritation. When you are ready to leave the house for your training appointment, wouldn't it be nice if you can find your gear, membership pass, and sneakers? If you recognize this to be the cause of stress, it means that it is time to get organized. The reason is, for once, not people but things and the ease of access, logic and ergonomics. Finding a logical storage place for your paraphernalia that is easy to get to makes sense. In a disorderly household, it is more difficult to find what you need or to move around. When I came home from the hospital, I was in a wheelchair. Soon you realize how important it is to combine the storage of items of the same category and to consider the ease of access. Take a close look at the environment where you spend time, from bathroom to kitchen, and see what can be done to improve the match with your ability. Ergonomic specialists can do that for you. They take the human factor into consideration when it comes to upgrading your environment and its components; a good design supports your self-sufficiency and safety. Streamlining your immediate surroundings with the help of friends or specialists will add to your feelings of well-being and independence and reduce stress.

Positive stress will speed up the way your mind works: faster and more clearly. In my work, I used to be fast and thorough in decision-making. Not long ago, my older son called for advice on his business, and for the first time in a long time, I noticed that my mental reflex of thinking rapidly through a wide range of options and considering all aspects and arguments was returning. He needed me to perform, and I loved it; I had not lost my touch.

In behavior, normal functioning is a flawed concept. It refers to some degree of deviation from what is perceived as the average by the majority. After a brain stroke, we may do things differently, which can lead to some questioning looks. Not only our values in life might have changed but also the way we interact with our environment. This may be reflected in our approach toward people, our rationale and emotions, and the way practical tasks are executed. The priority of the individual is first and foremost to regain satisfaction with his or her own new lifestyle as opposed to meeting the alleged norms of others—at least for as long as the norms and values of society are respected. The way of doing simple things in the outside world may take a lot more than the norm: making payments with a queue of impatient people behind you or delicately negotiating the stairs in a public building while everybody else is in a rush. It is important to ignore the sense of being pushed around by expectations and to do that with a smile.

Things take time, however long it takes. The impatience of others can introduce stress and anxiety, which in turn affects emotions and can make you feel awkward; which only makes things worse. A way of dealing with such situations is to avoid them in the first place—like staying away from the crowd in rush hour. Eliminating disturbing elements creates room for concentration. Without interference, to carry out one thing at a time, even with brittle functioning, can be a pleasure... even after a stroke. And that is what it is all about.

In the context of rehabilitation, my definition of the handling of negative stress provides an indication of the overall ability to deal with mental pressure.

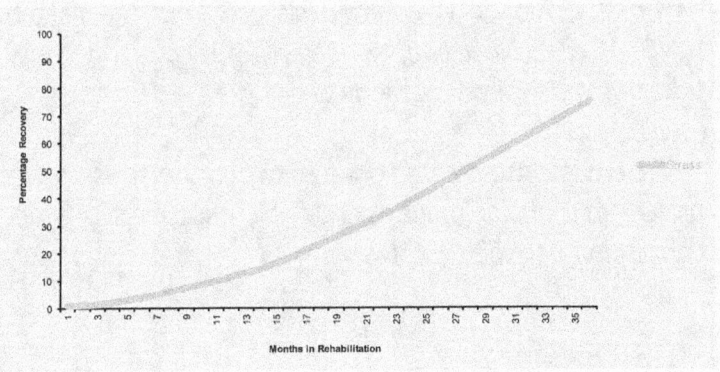

Figure 9. Stress Handling

The skill to deal with the impact of stress returned slowly after a long period of marginal advance. lit took approximately two years to recover one-third of my defenses against stress and to restrain the emotions unleashed by anxiety. During that time, I resided in the sheltered environment of my home or in one of the hospitals. Improvements were in small steps and hardly measurable. Nevertheless, there was a noticeable move forward over the long term. Stress is a normal part of our lives, and it could well be that my progress during the first years was slow due to my limited exposure to the forces of the outside world. Less seclusion could have reduced the stimulus to relearn more rapidly.

In the beginning, there is, of course, the fragile feeling of being secure. That can be due to a lack of reference and possible shortcomings in balance, vision, and speech. Those limitations play a big role in life and undermine your initial capacity. The real upswing did not start until core medical and physical areas showed clear signs of recovery. Nowadays, I rate my stress-handling ability as acceptable. Not to discourage anybody, but the golden rule is that the last twenty percent of recovery typically takes as much time as the first eighty.

There is close resemblance between the stress curve and the graph for multitasking, which suggests a direct correlation between the two.

Multitasking

Some people would argue that the ability of multitasking is genetically determined, and that because I am male, the topic would be irrelevant. The deep-rooted belief that women are better at multitasking than men has yet to be confirmed. All empirical evidence seems to support the idea that both genders are equal in their ability to multitask. However, the outcome of the battle between sexes may not matter. Our multitasking ability seems to be highly overrated and superficial. A core limitation of the brain is the inability to concentrate on two things at once.

Originally, the term multitasking comes from the computer world. It was associated with machines that could execute different instructions simultaneously. Researchers distrust the human ability to truly multitask: "When people say they can do better, they are deluding themselves." Their argument is backed up by studies revealing that the execution of tasks which we are carrying out compete for attention by the brain. Apparently our brain cannot focus on one thing while doing the other.

Multitasking, or actually the ability to toggle our attention between different tasks, allows us to deal with a mixture of different operations even though our consciousness is unable to focus on each of them concurrently. Time delays and errors can negatively affect the quality of our actions. Constantly switching focus is not always efficient or safe.

In most countries, it is forbidden to use a mobile phone whilst driving. The reason is due to the lack of full attention to the traffic and the lag in reaction time due to the change of one's concentration from talk to traffic. It is better to be safe than sorry; a split second delay in braking can be catastrophic.

Writing about one subject and simultaneously having a serious conversation on another unrelated topic creates a conflict in the ability to communicate efficiently. There will be a noticeable delay in our writing or replies while there is a higher chance of making mistakes due to insufficient concentration. The effect is blamed on neural interference among tasks; in this case, word and speech.

Rather than working things in parallel, we seem to act in order. Normally, our ability to switch between activities is incredibly fast. So rapid, that it is perceived as real multitasking. Nonetheless, as the multiplicity of tasks become more complex or unfamiliar, it takes us noticeably longer to regain concentration. Disruptions make the processing of information more cumbersome. Importantly, finishing a task may become more time consuming because of an increased number of mistakes that need to be fixed. To dismiss attempts at multitasking may be the wise thing to do.

After the stroke, I could no longer deceive myself or others; I had become mentally and physically slow. I do not believe that my intelligence had suffered, but my level of comprehension was falling behind. I would tilt at even the slightest sense of people confusing that with stupidity. Brain-training exercises showed that my little computer still worked. It was the tempo of understanding of what was asked of me, or what was happening in my surroundings, that caused delays in my response. Encouragingly, the ability to concentrate is better as we get older; it becomes easier to focus and block out interruptions. Is there a growing strength to compensate for an increasing weakness in order to maintain a healthy balance? I decided to experiment with single-tasking.

Many people in my surrounding perceived my quiet stance as being inflexible. In a way, they were right but for the wrong reasons. A spontaneous change of plans was suddenly no longer in the cards. Impulsiveness had left me. To my defense, there is a difference between "unwilling-and-able" and "willing-and-unable." I would place myself in the latter category. The inability to flip on a coin was a direct result of the stroke. When the mind is dawdling in gathering a response to demands from its surroundings, it is frustrating and tiring to deal with disruptions. One way or another, my choices, and therefore my flexibility, were restricted by the capability to manage stress, distribute my energy, react, and coordinate a response. I used to be able to serve everybody around me. Undisturbed by interruptions, I would participate in a vivid debate or address a myriad of subjects seemingly simultaneously. Now, a sluggish reaction time had undermined my assertiveness. It took longer to digest what was said, consider my options, and bring up my viewpoints. I was an easy target in discussions with those who don't take prisoners

In my previous life as a professional in the IT business, I had been operating at peak performance for many years.

I was used to dealing with an endless number of decisions, opinions, and strategies; from reviewing technical specifications to making policy, it was all in a day's work. Over time, my ability to rapidly switch from one topic to another had matured extremely well. It helped that I had the good fortune to grow with the company and knew the business inside out, which made dealing with the managerial topics a routine. To get the job done, some prerequisites were crucial: time and task management, stress management, and the allocation of undisturbed time to deal with complex tasks that needed all my concentration.

Making time to think, plan, and undertake intricate tasks improves efficiency and accuracy. This proved to be true in my work but also in my hobby of building model boats. As with many things, their beauty lies in the sum of the details; the satisfaction of doing a quality job is a reward by itself. When it comes to having a choice between doing a good job in the privacy of my concentration or creating a half-fledged product under the influence of constant interruptions, the decision is an easy one. It makes me happier to devote my attention to finishing a single project, or a number of smaller but similar tasks, than switching between unrelated activities. Working in an unstructured fashion is not me.

It all started to make sense. The time it takes to toggle your attention back and forth increases drastically when the interruptions miss any logical relation. The gap between scribbling down a shopping list while discussing dinner plans is small compared to writing a formal letter and trying to keep up a conversation on a totally different subject. Shifting activity is believed to be a two-step process. According to scientists, the unconscious has to drop the present task first before it can allocate system resources to a new mission. The bigger the dissimilarities in perception, thought, and action, the longer it takes to adjust. Even though we are only looking at a fraction of a second per switch, it starts to add up. It can be very difficult to regain full concentration on the main task. These days, an overdose of mental intrusions throws me totally off track.

Eventually, I got to know the new me. My reactions had changed. The cause was partially due to physical and mental limitations, but many were self-induced to protect my feelings. A major obstacle was dealing with mistakes that resulted from a lack of concentration. Noticing things going wrong was the same as declaring myself incompetent. Witnessing my own failure led to anxiety, and stress handling was one of my weakest points.

Directing my focus on one thing only, by consciously blocking out everything else, made me perform a lot better. It was a pleasure to complete a task less clumsily, with growing self-confidence, and in the absence of stress. The single-tasking approach had a positive impact on my well-being. A change in conduct asks for consideration by the surroundings. Without an explanation, the new behavior is easily perceived as inflexible, egocentric, or even antisocial. The change is not in character though, but purely practical. To eliminate any basis for misunderstanding and still stick to my outsets, I would simply respond to interruptions by showing that I was busy, plead for time to finish the current task, or ask to do another thing first. As long as I come back to the subject later, there is usually no harm done.

The impact of rapid task switching on everyday life is enormous. It seems to have become a constantly present phenomenon. Dropping out of the quest for alleged efficiency and productivity is considered contrary behavior in today's society. Then again, the person who lives by paying partial attention only ends up trading quantity for quality. That would not be fulfilling enough for me. Once distractions from the object of focus by irrelevant thoughts or my environment were eliminated, my days became less complicated. That included the need to stop interrupting myself.

My life in the fast lane is over, but there are no regrets. What bothers me is being pushed on the defensive. Stronger than ever, I suddenly noticed the increasing lack of respect that many people have for somebody's privacy. Who has not tried to relax with a good book but never managed to finish the open page? It is inconsiderate of people to barge in and expect you to drop everything and abruptly change your focus. It may take some time to learn how to best arm yourself against those cold intrusions.

Everything has its time and place. Finding a new balance between single-tasking and multitasking was influenced by many deficiencies; the ability to deal with the stress outweighs them all. It is difficult to keep up with the demands from society when forced to block out external impulses and place your own interest first. In the early period, there was no real choice; it was a matter of survival. My relearning required undivided attention down to every detail. My performance needed so much concentration that it was impossible to allow people or events to interrupt my action planning, thoughts, and execution. Absent-mindedly pouring a cup of coffee would result in a mess. As my ability to deal with stress improved, slowly some of the multitasking capability returned at a superficial level. I became better at handling interruptions or talks that were in line with my current activity. As long as there was an overlap with my focus and attempts, I would be able to incorporate comments and suggestions into my operation and deal with them smoothly but in an unhurried manner. When studying a travel guide, talking about which sites to visit, planning the day, and making notes on a map: all must be done simultaneously.

These days I am back to multitasking for simple and related tasks. For all that are complex and those that are unrelated, I stick to single-tasking out of convenience. I appreciate the pleasure of fulfilling a task properly more than ever before. It adds that extra bit of satisfaction to the job.

In the context of rehabilitation, my definition of multitasking provides an indication of the ability to smoothly switch between tasks and thus create the perception of paying full attention to impulses from the surroundings.

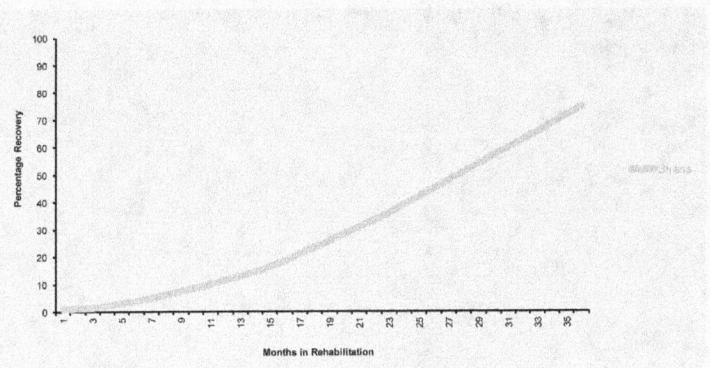

Figure 10. Multitasking

Effortlessly switching from task to task is part of everyday life. Without that ability, it is easy to become isolated from society. The challenge is to find the right balance between the personal satisfaction found in the privacy of one's own concentration and opening up to social interaction. The first two years after the stroke, my behavior was very much closed. Born out of necessity, single-tasking prevailed in all my doings, and anything that would defocus my attention was dismissed with a kind but stringent remark. It took time for my environment to accept the need to behave like that. I am grateful for their patience.

Today, I am much more at ease with alternating between subjects and tasks. Consciously, I limit multitasking to related themes and topics that are insignificant enough to be given my partial attention. My reaction is not as fast as I would like it to be, but my flexibility, as well as the feel of social integration, has drastically improved. I expect that my progress will continue to rise evenly over the years.

Brain Workout

Surprisingly enough brain training comes last in the line of therapies. It strikes me as odd. You get a brain stroke and everybody neglects the obvious.

Until recently, I was too busy with my focus on fitness training; active exercise of the brain stopped not far short from doing Sudokus and keeping up with the intricacies of daily routines. In the beginning of recovery, there are probably more pressing matters to address. Obviously, one's speed of interpretation is not a high priority for medical specialists when you have to learn to swallow, walk, and see properly again. Their first aim is to get you into the medical safe zone and help you to become self-sufficient. Thereafter, not a single therapist ever hinted at exploring the field of brain training; my being a bit slow was not their worry.

Brain training is a do-it-yourself job. I am glad that I took the initiative myself. I was hooked as soon as I experienced the positive effects. Common sense tells me that brain training must be something that you cannot start early enough.

Just consider the benefits to key areas of mental recovery such as stress handling, multitasking, concentration, and coordination. Rather than working toward recovery sequentially, it is something to do in parallel with physically- or medically-orientated tasks. Mental exercises can be done in bed, in your favorite chair, or on the beach and does not require more than some undisturbed time. An hour per day and the joy of working your brain in privacy will quickly yield results.

My habit of doing Sudokus with my morning coffee in the garden had become an innocent addiction. My brain slowly awakened under the already pleasant warmth of a Spanish daybreak. It was a simple luxury and a nice and quiet moment to myself with no stress, no talking, no physical inconveniences to concern myself with, and nobody but myself to judge my performance. In a matter of months, my capability to solve the numeric puzzles increased hugely; the simplest ones effortlessly and only limited by my speed of writing; the complex ones, solved before my morning coffee would have time to get cold. The progress and the joy of a private moment got me on the track of brain training.

Not long after coming out of rehabilitation, I took on simple domestic tasks: paying bills, booking airline tickets, or planning long-distance car travel. After a bit of frustration, I could take pride in mastering the re-entry into the digital world. The Internet simplified my daily life tremendously. It provided me with e-mail, daily news from all over the globe, the state of world economics, and in-depth analyses. The Internet is an active medium as opposed to TV. E-mails give you the opportunity to stay in touch with friends in a way that allows you to follow your own pace. By the end of the day, nobody can tell how long it took to compose the message. It provided me with the means of communication without the stress of making a telephone call with a raspy voice. It bought me time to be precise and thoughtful without the recipient's ever knowing the efforts.

Communication in black and white is less pardoning than oral. Verbally, you have the luxury to immediately correct a misinterpretation or elaborate on a topic. When the brain is too slow to intercept a mistake or your speech misses out on using the appropriate intonation, things you say may well become a liability. Long conversations were tiring; the attention level was not easy to uphold. The pros and cons of written over verbal communication change with your level of mental recovery. One thing suffices: written communication is prone to a higher degree of logic and accuracy. Subsequently, writing creates an extra stimulus for the brain.

When a good friend asked me to write a business plan, I gladly accepted. It was a challenge of my old professional skill: a mix of sales and marketing garnished with assumptions and numbers. It took me time to mull over the concept, consider all aspects of his ambition, appeal to investors, and put prose and revenues to it. While it took me longer than anticipated, the result was that once my brain eventually warmed up, I found a piece of my old self back. It was a motivating task; my brain had not given up on me. I was on my way back.

My creative talent has always been biased toward applying logic. Photography is as close as it gets to artistic imaging. A camera appeals to me with its shutter speeds and diaphragms and a tripod from which to carefully compose a classical picture. The dominance of the left side of my brain over the artistic right is above all reflected in my meager feel for rhythm and music, not that I have attempted to develop a talent for it either. The gift had come naturally to the rest of the family, and I was no match for them, so I did not bother. We all tend to focus on what we do best. What I learned about the brain made me decide to give it one final try. Who knows which hidden talent I possess: no pain, no gain.

The effects of a brain injury after a stroke can be extensive. I have been lucky enough to experience only moderate effects on my cognitive functions and emotions. Many of the possible disorders are much graver and require specialized therapy. Depending on the area and extent of the damage, someone suffering from aphasia may be able to speak but not write or vice versa. Fortunately, it is not the result of deficits in intellect or a cognitive disorder. Family and friends may notice a change in character and emotion. There may be signs of depression, self-overestimation, an easy outbreak in anger, or rapid changes in emotion.

The cognitive performance of the brain is the function most frequently affected by a stroke. As a result, the outward appearance of people who experienced brain injury is often much older than they really are. The manifestation of the disorder is frequently experienced by a lack of comprehension within a commonly accepted time frame. The mind seems to have lost the ability to perceive and understand. New situations constantly call upon our pool of knowledge and apply that to a practical understanding. What if our intellect does not readily seem to grasp the meaning or importance of something? It could be in the immediate understanding of text, verbal communication, a situation, or image. Without ample time to really comprehend what you just experienced, it is easy to be considered slow. Your intelligence, the use of stored information in the brain, and the application of it in finding the correct approach is not at fault. It is just a matter of speed. Fortunately, the reaction time is something that you can improve by brain training. A little bit of patience by the outside world can resolve what is left.

Slow cognitive performance makes you a dangerous driver. It directly affects your response time. I realized the effects en route to Malaga airport in Spain. Huge billboards along the highway advertised building projects and golf resorts. Under, say, thirty miles per hour, I could take my time as a passenger to study the lush greens and pools that were promised and would have time to take in the name of the agency. At sixty miles per hour, all of that information was wasted on me. At best, I could recall that it was about some kind of complex, but do not bother to ask me about the details, however compressed the marketing message might have been.

Imagine a busy crossing, with multiple lanes and traffic lights and constantly moving traffic, pedestrians, and bicycles and the time it takes to process all that changing information in order to be safe to others and yourself. Brain training improves your spatial insight and the time it takes to recognize patterns and improve reaction time. Benchmarks by drivers' licensing authorities may assist in the consideration of whether you should get behind the wheel or continue to enjoy the ride as a passenger.

Over time, I have overcome many of my shock reactions. At least I suppress them better. As a car passenger, my reaction to the sudden emergence of other traffic used to drive my chauffeur crazy. An unexpected noise can make me freeze in anxiety as if a firecracker were going off behind my back. I believe that my strong emotional reflexes boil down to the same theme: not being able to determine the source of an event fast enough and therefore, being unable to control my reaction.

The way the brain functions is as fascinating as it is unknown. It is still largely unmapped territory to neurologists, psychologists, and many other scientists. Numerous faculties made it their study object. The associated research is extremely broad and ranges from behavioral science to artificially mimicking intelligence. In the context of rehabilitation after a brain injury, the focus of the patient is fortunately limited to practicalities, as opposed to requiring a theoretical understanding, to improve the efficient functioning of the brain.

In the thirteenth century, Thomas Aquinas had already divided the study of human behavior into two broad categories: the cognitive experience—how we have learned to know the world—and our emotions. Thinking, art, a technical invention, effective communication, ambition, or concentration—they are all results of our brain activity. All are in need of evaluation, integration, and initiation of information in a certain framework. It is amazing what the brain can achieve. After hundreds of years, the cognitive processes, such as memory, association, language, and problem solving, remain to be regarded as brain functions, although the division between cognitive and emotion is now challenged. Nevertheless, cognition is generally accepted to mean the process of thought and is a unique property of human beings.

A distinctive feature of the brain is the ability to mold itself from inception to a point of maturity at which time it forms the stable inner calm of the individual. That stability reduces the impact of external influences on a person's behavior. It makes a person reliable and predictable in the way he or she acts and performs. The quality to adapt is reduced over the years but remains a characteristic that is capable of further modification in case of damage or old age and through repetitive exercises.

Another unique characteristic of the brain in case of damage is the ability to reroute the flow of signals between neurons. Unless it is a major neurological information highway, the brain will explore secondary routes or build bridges to the information it seeks. This ability is limited to small damages only but worth treasuring for the gift it is. Repetitive brain training is alleged to stimulate the repair process and hence aid our cognitive functions. Nurturing the possession of these qualities should not be neglected—which speaks in favor of brain training.

Brain training may help to increase your flexibility and multitasking. After a stroke, things often do not go as smoothly as they used to; simple daily routines require a lot of concentration. The mind is focused on a particular task and is so preoccupied with planning, that it is difficult to break away from the task at hand; there is no room to address an unpredicted request. It may be that I am on my way out the door to dump the garbage and find it difficult to change my bearing when asked to collect some other things as well. The course and act are premeditated. Deviation from the plan interferes with achieving my objective. In such a situation, I would take the easy route and would rather walk twice. That same lack of flexibility creates stress. It may be that you have intended to do things in a certain sequence. Perhaps you are cooking dinner for friends and have all the steps well organized; all ingredients are pre-cut, measured, and lined up. All goes well until something unexpected happens; the sauce boils over. A lack of reaction time and flexibility will probably cause a slight panic at the stove. The dinner evening, however, does not have to be spoiled. By now people should understand your poor crisis behavior and not be offended for their serving to be put on hold when told, "One second please. Let me finish this first and clean up the mess."

Hospitalization over a longer period takes its toll on the brain. When living in a small and safe environment which is controlled by a team that is dedicated to your well-being, the brain gets lazy when deprived of mental activity. Just like the loss of strength due to a lack of physical exercise, the neurons take a vacation. Hold on to your brain condition as well as possible, and strive to improve it. Try to attend to more than undemanding routines, and make time to stimulate your brain functions. Training the command center of the brain requires concentration, precision, and endless repetition. Conversely, it is not a gigantic or unpleasant task.

As a student, I had always enjoyed the noble game of chess, and after many years, my interest awakened again when I found a box of pieces on a bookshelf in the community room. The game requires spatial insight, strategy, and forward thinking. All of those aspects need concentration. It is a fantastic way to stimulate the brain with the luxury of your opponent thinking you're being slow for thoughtful contemplation of your moves. For me, it is chess; others may prefer another kind of board game or enjoy playing cards. They have one thing in common: silently, they train the brain and encourage socializing.

Over the years, our mental processes typically lose some of their efficiency. Further weakening of the cognitive functions comes at a bad time if one wants to undo that. With age, reversing the process will require some extra effort; that work can be enjoyable, even competitive. Before long, you may well find a buddy who is curious enough to join the fun. Most designs of the exercises have that effect on people.

As a family tradition, the jigsaw puzzle came onto the table over Christmas. As the family members trickled in for the celebration, young and old would join in the team effort to complete the undertaking. It is a very social task; people work at the puzzle on and off, chat, drink, laugh, and update each other on the latest family gossip. After months of rehabilitation, you start to see a training opportunity in almost everything. When desperate to act on automatic pilot without analyzing every step of the way, it may be time to recognize the feeling as a signal to take some time off and enjoy the holidays for what they are.

When my eyesight had sufficiently improved, I took up reading again. A good novel crafts a world that is only limited by the boundaries of your imagination. Books can create one of the easiest brain travels. If only for that reason, I was relieved that my eyesight had recovered. Reading is yet another way to stimulate your cognitive brain capacity.

One does not have to be computer literate or even own a PC to get started with brain training. There are numerous magazines and puzzle books in almost every language and in universal numbers to challenge the brain for a lifetime. On the other hand, worth mentioning is the Nintendo handheld game computer. The toy is operated by touch screen and stylus, and it supports voice recognition. The good news for the older generation is that one does not have to be experienced at playing computer games. Dr. Ryuta Kawashima is the brain behind the game programs that will tease the adult mind. His work contains a collection of simple daily exercises that help to stimulate the brain.

I found my favorite brain-training site on the Internet. The website was free upon registration. They offered a wide range of exercises in faculties such as calculus, language, memory, and spatial insight, as well as theme parks with sports, travel, literature, finance, etc. Course levels with exams at bachelor, master, and the PhD level provided a structured approach. The personal scores are measured by the mix of right and wrong and time. The latter adds the element of working under the stress of a ticking clock. By rating the combination of speed and cognitive performance simultaneously, it provides a nice tool to measure your degree of comprehension. Additional statistics allowed me to assess my personal performance against the average score of the other students. It is always nice to know how you stand up in the crowd.

For some years now, computer specialists and clinicians from many different countries and companies have joined forces to advance and promote "virtual rehabilitation." Experts have built tools based on advanced computer game technology and virtual reality to help people to recover from strokes, cognitive disorders, and more. Game-like exercises might well motivate patients who may otherwise lack the interest in the traditional rehabilitation regime. It holds the promise to fit the needs of this day and age. Video game technology has ceased to be simply a recreational tool; with, for instance the Nintendo Wii sports, you can set up a virtual gym and neural practice in your own living room; even a golf course or ski slope will fit.

It may be useful to look at the hundreds of titles of action games at your local computer store. They provide a form of entertainment that will test your reaction time and coordination. Not everybody will be too thrilled about computer games entering their lives, but it may be worthwhile; try it, and see how you experience gaming. Not all games have a violent mission; there are enough games around with a playful but serious educational touch to choose from.

Whatever brainteaser works for you; remember, it has to be diverse and fun. However valuable it may be, approach brain training as a game. Build it up slowly. It is more motivating to get an easy pass from one level up to the next than to be thrown back right from the start.

Epilogue

Shoots can grow to become big trees, but once a plant, always a plant. I have never been that plant—neither in intensive care nor at any other time on my sickbed, however slow my mind or fragile my life might have been. I resent the qualification; it is negative, inaccurate, and holds nothing for the future. I am human and have a brain. I have intellect, emotions, memories, and willpower.

In casual conversations, it was easy for people to describe my condition after the stroke as a "vegetable" when trying to make their point. I know it is nothing more than an innocent cliché, but the analogy mattered to me. In my presence, people knew not to use the expression. I had survived, and I was determined to get my life back. I was not going to end up on the windowsill to be watered, if not forgotten, or talked-down to. For the rest of my life, I could be in need of permanent nursing. That worrisome outlook was dismissed from day one; my focus was on reconditioning mind and body for a new and rewarding lifestyle. It was an open-ended endeavor. I was determined not to give in without a fight. My battle strategy was based on trust, perseverance, and patience. Like a newborn, I relearned the most basic skills.

Calling a brain stroke a "valuable experience" is nonsense. It is just another cliché. Life does not come without thorns. Yes, I learned a lot, but I never asked for the insights, and it has cost me my dreams. I was happy with my life as it was. With the experience, not my values but my attitudes have changed. I have become milder, more subtle in ventilating my opinions, and an empathic listener, but I became less forgiving to negativism that undermined my goals. I could hardly control my emotions when a fellow patient kept complaining about his misfortune: "I used to run up and down the stairs. I can't do that anymore." His nagging was poison to my motivation. What mattered was today and, the future, not the past. What I could or could not do was water under the bridge. I was grateful to be alive.

The reasons for my early retirement had been diverse; many of my generation had passed away, which made me fear for my health, and I wanted more out of life than work; I wanted things that would be difficult to realize as a pensioner. Getting a stroke was pure irony, a stroke of bad luck.

I submit myself to the unruffled beauty outdoors: white and frosty during the Norwegian winter, the sky full of stars, continuous daylight during the summer, and the warmth of Spain. I appreciate things in life more than before. None is materialistic: a short ferry crossing over the Oslo fjord, exuberant autumn colors, or watching the flow of people from a terrace at the port. A greater consciousness has taken over. There is no reason to feel sorry for myself.

I look out over Vigeland Park from behind a small desk on the veranda and observe, reflect, and think; I meditate.

Memory associations form a path like domino bricks as I reflect on my acts as a human being. Already early in the morning, the park is full of joggers of all ages. Although I have never met the man, one of them I know so well. He is in his seventies. Months ago, I spotted him for the first time; his feet dragged noisily through the gravel. Now, I watch him with a smile; his tempo is up and steady. Rehabilitation is not medical but physical and mental. The duration is measured in months or years, if not the rest of one's life. Success is for the strong-minded. It requires patience, persistence, and attitude.

Rehabilitation is a choice you make. It is not something that you passively submit to. You take a stance and act-and-react with an iron discipline to the demands. It is all about attitude: a mindset with a complex mix of beliefs, feelings, values, and dispositions. A positive attitude will keep you on track. Dismiss negative forces that create doubt or self-pity. You have to take command. Nobody but you can reshape your life. You cannot live the life of others or their expectations. The more proud you are of your achievements, the greater the satisfaction with your life.

There are no failures in rehabilitation unless you allow them to undermine your attitude. Accept failures as stepping-stones to improvement. Learn from them, and they will show new directions for growth. Awareness creates the opportunity to make intelligent choices regarding your self-improvement strategy. As you pay attention to the messages of mind and body, you get better and wiser by the day.

You can have a rewarding life without winning a Nobel Prize. A rewarding lifestyle is the materialization of one's ambition. How it turns out depends on the drive of the individual, which in turn is the sum of attitude and one's search for happiness. For starters, try living a life that gives personal satisfaction through doing the right things the right way. It may be in your own privacy or publicly, in your hobby, the arts, science, or community. A rewarding life often starts with sharing your talents, skills, or knowledge. Consistently making small contributions will add up to something to be recognized for. I went back to basics and shared the things I did best and people acknowledged me for it. Despite my limitations, I could add value to the lives of people around me.

My relationship to others has a big impact on the way I experience quality of life. I realized that when the ones I loved visited me in the hospital and reflected on our memories. I enjoyed it then and even more so now. Investing more of my time in personal and professional relationships has strengthened my sense of living a rewarding life.

Happiness is an agreeable feeling of well-being which assumes being at peace with yourself. People are all unique, and what is valid for one does not have to be true for somebody else. Even so, there are a number of common denominators in reaching a state of happiness.

Happiness is driven by positive emotions that relate to what lies ahead of us, behind us, or in the present. Optimism, hope, and trust are emotions of the future. Satisfaction, pride, contentment, and inner peace are positive emotions from the past. The longer the list of positive experiences, the more valuable the memory; it adds stability to sentiment. That is not necessarily true for the short flashes of superficial pleasure in daily life; it is easy come, easy go. Overeagerly chasing stimuli, without having confidence in the future, is not enough to produce a long-lasting feel of happiness. On the other hand, when devoting yourself to others consistently, it will create a sustainable feel of happiness.

Like attitude, my search for happiness implied making choices. The stroke had drastically changed the circumstances, which called for a new look at the way I would live my life. The obvious step to take was to radically dismiss all negative forces and to avoid situations that I could not step up to. It meant detaching myself from negative sentiments such as pessimism, discontent, and shame that could undermine my feelings of well-being. I could not let them influence my reactions or recovery. Conversely, I used my energy on optimism, gratification, and pride. I claimed the freedom to positively discriminate people and set my own itinerary. The approach narrowed but deepened my social life. Now, I could give undivided attention to the people who mattered. Secondly, I will always be grateful, not for the stroke, but for what I am today and for the people who love and care for me. I know no bitterness. There is no blame, just gratitude and the power of pride. Last, but not least, I took control over my future. Now, a few years after the stroke, I am still busy recovering, or better said, relearning.

Dorthe is back to work in the fashion business. Now it is my turn to be the caregiver. Solidarity starts early in the morning with making a pot of fresh coffee. During the day, I putter around, attend to domestic and social chores, do the shopping, and write. The old Jag is parked in the garage; I am hardly behind the wheel. The driver's seat is Dorthe's post; polishing is my meditative work: wax on, wax off. We exclusively travel by car for our joy and the journeys are as pleasurable as the destinations. The trips through continental Europe and Scandinavia gave us inspiration, quality time, and privacy.

I look at the stars and realize how little I know about the night sky. It is time to work on my knowledge of basic astronomy; I want to get to know what seems so close. Life has so many different dimensions.

Appendix 1 – Personal Economy

Sudden hospitalization and a long recovery process can have a big impact on the personal economy and domestic administration, particularly if the patient runs his or her own company or is self-employed. It may be necessary to transfer the day-to-day management to a business partner or a well-trusted employee or to hire an interim manager to ensure continuity. Without insurances, it may be difficult to maintain income or continue the business. How to act in a worst-case scenario is best considered before things go sour, but most people put off such an unpleasant task until it is too late. It could then be up to the caregiver to make the best out of it. Delegate specialist tasks; for one, because there might be little time left to attend to them properly. The tasks of a caregiver are already demanding enough without the extra workload and added stress. Technically, physically, or psychologically, it may be too much to handle.

Not all tasks related to the economy at home have to be that complex. When employed by a larger corporation, it tends to be a bit easier. Open communication with the manager and human resources specialist can give the caregiver more insight into the short- and long-term implications. You may find more than a willing ear. Do not be afraid to ask for active support to deal with the intricacies. The counselor at the hospital may be of assistance when it comes to understanding issues with respect to health insurance coverage or the procedures related to welfare and disability.

There will be many domestic administrative tasks that need attention: bills to pay, housing to be secured, taxes to be filed, and maybe investments to manage. A family member or accountant could help. To avoid potential problems with delegating finances or running a company for the interim, I recommend drafting a formal agreement in which you give the power of attorney to someone and specify the limits of authority. This is not because of a lack of trust, but to make certain you are involved when it comes to large sums of money or to ensure that major business decisions are not made over the head of the patient or partner. For the other party, the agreed boundaries will help to set the expectations and serve as operating guidelines.

Appendix 2 – Statistics

Statistics[1] for a brain stroke make horrifying reading. It is not something people like to look into unless confronted with the situation; neither did I. In a way, my wife and I are glad not to have fully understood how serious the circumstance of the hospitalization was. I now realize how lucky I am to be what and where I am today. A word of comfort: statistics are anonymous, and there is only one of you. With conviction, hard work, and a bit of luck, it is possible to beat the average.

The scary news is that brain strokes are the number one cause of adult disability and the second leading cause of death worldwide and third in the US. The other infamous top two are heart disease and cancer. A change in lifestyle

---

1 Source compilation (2007-2009): American Heart Association (AHA), American Stroke Association (a division of the AHA), American Society of Interventional and Therapeutic Neuroradiology, American Brain Attack Coalition, Centers for Disease Control, The University Hospital New Jersey, National Institute of Neurological Disorders and Stroke (NINDS), National Stroke Association, Centre for Chronic Disease Prevention and Control, Canadian Cardiovascular Society, Heart and Stroke Foundation of Canada, World Health Organization.

after a stroke can make a big difference for one's future when considering the outlook of a recurring stroke. A quarter of the victims have another stroke within the first five years.

The numbers paint a nasty picture. According to the World Health Organization, fifteen million people suffer from a stroke worldwide each year. The impact on human life is enormous: a third recover, a third are permanently disabled, and a third die.

Brain strokes affect more than seven hundred thousand individuals annually in the United States. Well over half a million of these are first attacks; the remainder are recurrent. More than four million people in the United States have survived a brain stroke and are living with the after-effects. Somehow, brain strokes affect four out of five families over the course of a lifetime. According to the American Heart Association (AHA), someone suffers a stroke every forty-five seconds.

The incidence rate for a stroke of bad luck varies by gender, race, and age. Occurrences lie between fifty-nine to ninety-three victims per one hundred thousand people. Statistically, male African-Americans are the worst off. Numbers from the United States indicate that more than a third of stroke victims recover almost completely or sustain only minor deficiencies. Forty percent experience moderate to severe impairments. Ten percent will need permanent care in a nursing home. Fifteen percent do not make it. Bleeding into the brain due to a rupture of one of its blood vessels causes the so-called hemorrhagic stroke. It is the most severe. Although it accounts for only seven percent of all strokes, the fatality rate is over fifty percent. Of the survivors, approximately half suffer permanent disability.

Europe averages approximately 650,000 stroke deaths each year. In developed countries, the incidence of stroke is declining. This is largely due to efforts to lower blood pressure and a reduction of smoking. However, the overall rate of stroke remains high due to the aging of the population.

The estimate of the economic cost of stroke in the United States is a staggering forty-three billion USD annually. Of this amount, nearly two-thirds is for medical care and therapy. The indirect costs from a loss of productivity and other factors cover the remainder. The average cost of care for a patient up to three months after stroke is fifteen thousand USD. For ten percent of the patients, the cost of care for that period is more than double that. The direct costs of care for the first months is broken down to initial hospitalization (forty-three percent), rehabilitation (sixteen percent), physician costs (fourteen percent), hospital readmission (fourteen percent), and medications and other expenses (thirteen percent).

Appendix 3 - Timeline of Recovery

Month, location, and primary activity:

0–1   Ullevål Universitet Sykehus, Oslo, Norway.

      Intensive care and medical emergencies.

2–4   Diakonhjemmet Sykehus, Oslo, Norway.

      Medical treatment with the focus on nutrition and initial rehabilitation.

5–7   Sunnaas Rehabiliterings Sykehus, Nessodden, Norway.

      Dedicated first line rehabilitation.

8–9   Cato Rehabiliterings Senteret, Son, Norway.

      Dedicated second line rehabilitation.

10–17 At home. Oslo, Norway.

Vocal cord operation. Private rehabilitation. Voice therapy and personal training at SATS Fitness Centre. Mostly indoors.

18–33 Temporary move to Puerto Banus, Spain.

Private rehabilitation. Physical training at the Platinum Wellness and Fitness Centre. Mostly outdoors.

34-36 At home. Oslo, Norway.

Private rehabilitation. Physical training at Elixia Fitness Centre combined with outdoor activities. Return to society.

About the Author

Sebastiaan Bakker was born in Amsterdam, the Netherlands in 1951.

Educated as an engineer, he worked most of his professional life in a variety of executive management positions for an American Multinational in the IT sector until his early retirement in 2001. He prepared for living aboard a sailboat in the Mediterranean with his wife until he suffered a stroke in his brain stem, which wiped out nearly all of his physical and biological stability and life support systems.

Ironically, his decision for retirement was strongly related to the loss of his first wife to cancer and many colleagues and friends who died young or shortly after having reached their pension age. Now his world was once again turned upside down. In his book, he describes what it takes to come from a position where breathing was the only thing he was capable of, to his happiness three years later.

His focus is on the power of positive thinking in the rehabilitation process. The problem, other than understanding it, is not worth his energy; only the solution matters. From one day to another, he ventured into a new world where nothing could be taken for granted and all his functions required reprogramming. He found himself in a new job, one in which he would need all his professional experience mixed with optimism, motivation, a strong discipline, and self-management skills. Failure was no option.

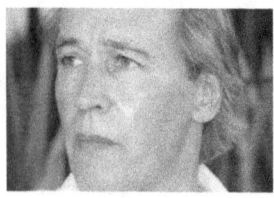 Practical examples give a unique insight, from medical recovery to the return to society, to patients as well as family and friends. Many readers can gain from the understanding that arises. Illustrations show the process of healing over time by key area: medical, mental, and physical. He found a new and rewarding lifestyle by overcoming the challenges of everyday life: step-by-step, day in, day out.

Embedded in his personal account are numerous hints and tips and points to consider. Rather than plain telling, the story triggers the imagination and makes it easier to recognize behavioral or physical symptoms. By doing so, the author hopes to reduce the struggle by other individuals who ended up in a similar situation and of those in their surroundings. The importance of the role of caregiver is intertwined with the story throughout the book and summarized in a dedicated chapter.